WARD ATTENDING:

THE FORTY-DAY MONTH

Lucy M. Osborn, M.D.
Professor, Department of Pediatrics
University of Utah School of Medicine

Neal Whitman, MPA, Ed.D.
Professor, Department of Family
and Preventive Medicine
University of Utah School of Medicine

epilogue by

Clifford J. Straehley, M.D.
Professor, Department of Surgery
John A. Burns School of Medicine

This book is dedicated to Dr. Anne Osborn, a consummate teacher ...and a consummate sister.

LO

This book is dedicated to Dr. Thomas L. Schwenk, a lifelong learner ...and a lifelong friend.

NW

Design and Production by

Rebecca M. Childs

CONTENTS

INTRODUCTION

This book is a result of collaboration between a doctor of medicine and a doctor of education. Both professions share the aim of helping others. Just as one can think of a medical interview as a theme-based conversation based upon the needs of a patient, similarly, one can think of an educational encounter as a theme-based conversation based on the needs of a learner.

This book is aimed at helping attending physicians who are challenged with the task of helping two groups of people at the same time: the patients admitted to their clinical service and the medical students and residents assigned to them. In many teaching hospitals, clinicians are asked to attend at least one month a year. When you attend, does it feel like a forty-day month?

We ask because many clinical teachers have told us that attending is one of the most difficult and demanding months of the year. With the approaches suggested in this book, the authors hope to reduce the stress of attending physicians and to optimize the learning of medical students and residents.

In asking you to think about your clinical teaching, we realize that you may not be rewarded for your teaching (Whitman and Roth 1990). Also, we recognize that teaching may not be one of your major responsibilities. Nevertheless, if you are reading this book, we assume that there is some desire to become a better teacher. As one assistant professor of medicine wrote, "I hope that the teacher trapped within this researcher's body may be eventually released" (Miller 1990).

The potential for improvement is underscored in the following not atypical scenarios:

> The attending is known for arriving late at morning report. Anticipating this, the admitting resident presents the most complicated patient first, hoping to finish before the attending arrives. The attending arrives in the middle of the presentation, makes a few critical comments, and leaves.

> During a medical student's lengthy presentation of every finding, including all the normals, every resident is paged out of the room at least once, so that by the end no one has heard the whole case. Then the attending and the medical student engage in a lengthy discussion and others look bored.

> At the end of morning report, the attending physician asks a chief resident what his future plans are and the two chat while others are impatient to start work rounds.

> Medical students and residents jiggle their beepers, hoping to avoid questions like "How was syphilis named?" or "Why are some organs paired?"

In developing ways to avoid these pitfalls, attending physicians should keep in mind that medical students and residents share responsibility for the educational outcomes of ward teaching. This partnership came to mind when we learned about a new inventory system used by some hospitals to save money, "just in time " operations. In these systems, one vendor fills all hospital orders, sometimes in small amounts, and delivers directly to departments what they need on a daily basis. It occurs to us that there is a "just in time" application to the learning process.

Sometimes, do we treat medical students and residents like warehouses where information can be stored for future use? Instead, we should recognize that learning is not a matter of filling a void with information. Optimal learning will occur when students and residents are ready to receive and use information. According to this view, the attending physician has to find out what is needed so that "just in time" learning can occur. But, just as the hospital supply company cannot anticipate the hospital's needs without hospital input, the attending physician cannot determine the learner's needs in a vacuum. A partnership is required so that what is needed is supplied in the right amount.

In the early nineteenth century, A. Bronson Alcott wrote, *"The true teacher defends his pupils against his own personal influence."* One interpretation of this statement is that a teacher should let students make their own mistakes - that's how they will learn! Another interpretation is that a teacher should use his* experience to protect students from making the same mistakes the teacher has made. In any case, attending physicians can and should do both . . . sometimes allowing medical students and residents to make their own mistakes and sometimes stopping them. Deciding which is the case requires judgment, and we believe that attending physicians will make better judgments if they and the ward team members view each other as partners. A lack of partnership is evident when decisions made by the ward team with the attending physician during morning report are changed at afternoon signout rounds with the chief resident without any consultations with the attending physician (Collins, Cassie, and Daggett 1978).

In chapters one and two, the role and responsibility of the attending physician in this partnership are addressed. In these chapters, the authors recognize that attending physicians have to balance the quality of patient care with learning opportunities for medical students and residents. In chapter three, the domains of learning are discussed in terms of knowledge, attitudes, and skills, and, in chapters four and five, the teaching of communication skills and communicating through the medical record are described.

---

* It should be noted at this point that teachers (and readers) are both male and female, of course. But, the text consistently uses the pronoun he (or his). Although the s/he (his/her) construction may help reduce bias, we feel that it makes awkward reading. Our intention is not to promote sex stereotyping, but simply to provide concise writing.

Now that medical students have left the classroom for the "application" environment, the teaching of procedures is addressed in chapter six, and, because of the attending physician's position at the top of the medical team, how to manage medical mistakes and how to assess and give feedback to medical students and residents are reviewed in chapters seven and eight. If there has been adequate feedback, medical students and residents will not be surprised by your evaluation of their performance, the subject of chapter nine.

Finally, we welcomed the contribution of a clinical teacher, who at the time of his retirement, offered his perspective. We hope that readers find Dr. Clifford J. Straehley's look backwards a stimulus to their looking forward. Being an attending physician is a challenging endeavor and, as the health care delivery system and medical education undergo change, new challenges can be expected.

In the Introduction to *Creative Medical Teaching,* (1990) Neal Whitman admitted that writing a book was presumptuous. One presumes to have something useful to say! In this book, Lucy M. Osborn and Neal Whitman presume to have something useful to say to attending physicians. To the degree that the reader gives and gets more out of being an attending physician, their confidence will be justified. They hope that we have not taken liberties with your time.

6 Ward Attending

CHAPTER 1

The Role of the Attending Physician

The process of learning the practice of medicine is very different from learning to be an accountant in that medical education cannot be separated from patient care. This means that teaching young doctors is a constant balancing act. How can you teach a medical student to care for a complicated medical problem and still ensure adequate care for the patient? How can an attending provide supervision, yet allow a resident enough independence to create a good learning environment?

Attending on hospital wards is one of the most challenging jobs facing physicians in academic centers today. In the past, the majority of medical training took place in hospital settings. Students and residents learned basic skills through caring for patients who were usually assigned to a "house service." Often, these were indigent patients who did not have a private physician directing their medical care.

Over the past twenty-five years medicine has changed dramatically. Many diseases that required hospitalization in the past are now readily treated on an outpatient basis. Changes in patient mix, length of stay, and reimbursement have resulted in making ward rotations a very different experience for students and residents. Generally, hospitalized patients are now much sicker than in years past. They are often quickly discharged to home care or other facilities. Because the financing of medical education is now greatly dependent upon clinical revenues, most patients will have an attending of record who is actively involved in the patient's clinical care.

All of these changes have made an impact upon the role of the attending and upon the relationship between attendings, residents, and students. One of the most difficult issues for both attendings and residents is the balance between independent resident decision making and attending control. The attending physician is responsible for the care given to the patient both ethically and medicolegally. Yet, the resident is the one who directly delivers the patient care. To learn the practice of medicine, the resident must accept responsibility for the care of the patient and must be allowed to make decisions regarding medical management. In addition, often the residents, not the attending physicians, directly supervise medical students. Thus, the attending is in the uncomfortable position of being responsible for the patient's care, but not truly being in control.

The dual responsibility of teaching trainees assigned to a ward and of supervising the care given to patients was identified in a study by Collins, Cassie and Doggett (1978) in which attending physicians viewed these responsibilities as inextricably entwined. Based on a variety of data sources, including questionnaires, interviews, and videotaped segments of ward rounds, they found a lack of definition regarding the purpose of ward rounds and a lack of planning for the educational component of rounds, leading to a situation in which neither patient care nor teaching were efficiently handled!

There are other factors that have added stress to this relationship. The issue of resident working hours places large constraints on the ability of residents to provide continuity of care for hospitalized patients. If continuity becomes the responsibility of the attending, the role of the resident is reduced, as is his learning experience. Another factor is the medicolegal environment. Recently there have been incidents in which residents have been sued separately from attendings in malpractice cases.

Although the dilemma is difficult, there are certainly means to address the problems. The purpose of this book is to outline methods that can assist attendings in creating a balance between their educational mission and their medical responsibilities. The following chapters will discuss the requisite leadership and management skills and teaching methods that can make the experience of attending rewarding for all concerned.

The key to successful attending is in the relationship that is formed between the attending and the students and residents. The smooth running of a ward team is dependent upon the leadership skills of the attending and the supervisory resident. Although mistakes and differences of opinion regarding management of patient care are inevitable, these can be minimized if the attending and the residents can follow some simple procedures. Good communication among all parties is essential. Explicit explanations of expectations for performance and a clear understanding of the roles of the various members of the ward team will enhance the functioning of each of the team members.

The most crucial element in avoiding problems is communication. The first procedure to be agreed upon should be a system of communication between the attending and the residents and students. Attendings are usually not present on the wards for a large portion of the day, while the residents are expected to be readily available to admit patients and to provide on-going observation and management. The most frequent complaint from attendings is that they are not informed regarding decisions for care or changes in the status of their patients.

The residents, on the other hand, complain that they are "used" by attendings who need their help with service requirements, but do not teach. Exchange of information is expected on morning rounds, but seldom are other communication systems explicitly defined. At a minimum, the supervisory resident should have ready access to the attending of record, either by telephone or by pager. It is then the responsibility of the attending to clearly state his expectations regarding communications. Discussions between the attending and supervisory resident should result in a list of circumstances that require consultation with the attending.

Although it seems a simple enough task for an attending to inform residents when he would like to be called, it is, in fact, quite difficult. Few attendings would choose to be called regarding routine laboratory tests, while every attending should be notified if there is an important change in a patient's condition. When critical management decisions hinge on the results of tests, the attending may wish to discuss the results with the resident as soon as tests have been completed. Important considerations in requesting that residents have on-going communication include the stability of the patient, the likely course of the patient's disease, social considerations, and the skills of the resident.

An attending's skills in evaluation of the patient and understanding the projected course of the illness are much greater than those of the residents. After ascertaining what the resident expects, it is wise for the attending to modify those expectations and explain when he would want to be contacted. For example, residents frequently miss signs of impending respiratory failure in young infants with bronchiolitis or reactive airway disease. The attending should communicate to the resident how he wishes the patient to be followed (*e.g.* frequent vital signs, following the pCO$_2$), under what circumstance he must be notified, and how he can be reached.

At the same time, the attending needs to be conscious of the "learning vector" proposed by Stritter (1986). This model is based on the assumption that clinical instruction can influence a learner's professional development in a linear or stepwise fashion. The amount of independence expected from the learner needs to be closely matched with the medical learner's skills and maturity.

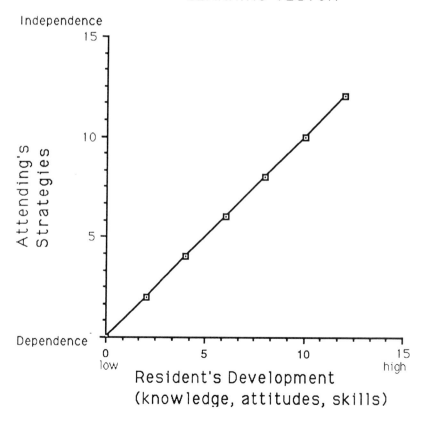

LEARNING VECTOR

In the medical environment, if the learner is given no guidance or supervision when he has only minimal skills, the result will be anxiety and fear rather than learning. On the other hand, if little independence is given to a mature learner, the result will be resentment, anger, and boredom. The only way that an attending can judge the learner's skills is through direct observation and close communications. Thus, at the beginning of an attending rotation, the attending may need to be in hourly contact with the supervisory resident. Once the attending is confident that the resident has the skills necessary to ensure the safety and appropriate care of patients, fewer telephone consultations will be required. It is also wise to arrange several times during the day when the resident can update the attending regarding the patients and the functioning of the team.

A different model is described by Kenneth Iserson in his discussion of the educational and ethical dilemmas of supervising physicians in training and the delicate balance between training physicians and the responsibilities for ensuring good patient care (1988). He suggests that a model of "credentialing and available supervision" be established. This would allow graded responsibility for students and protection of patient welfare, but would require attendings to be on-site and constantly available. Such a system would require that "a specific (1) knowledge base, (2) mastery of skills, and (3) master of problem solving and decision-making skills..." be defined.

Prior review or on-site supervision of decisions or procedures by a credentialed physician would be required for all students and residents who had not yet been credentialed to perform a given task. The advantages of such a system is that it would enhance preceptor-trainee interactions and ensure immediate feedback. The disadvantage is that, with the current organization of our medical schools and residency programs, this model may not be practical. Until the day that faculty are relieved of all other responsibilities during attending rotations, constant, on-site supervision by faculty is not feasible. Unless there were specific programs to train and credential all supervisory residents, the faculty would essentially be required to take the place of the supervisory resident, so that this experience would not be available to physicians-in-training.

Clearly defined procedures for communication facilitate the ability of the attending and supervisory resident to establish and maintain their roles and those of other members of the ward team. The next essential procedure is an explicit discussion with all team members about the goals and objectives for resident and student education and for patient care.

The overall goal of inpatient rotations is no different than that of medical school education and residency training in general, *i.e.* for students and residents to become competent physicians. Certainly, many of the learning objectives for students and residents on inpatient rotations are ones that apply to their general education. Other objectives are more specific to the setting. One of the ways to approach teaching is to analyze each situation and define the specific skills and tasks that are best taught in that setting. This enables the teacher both to concentrate his effort and limit the content so that the energy and thought expended result in a maximal learning experience.

Consideration needs to be given to the skills that students at various levels must develop that can best be learned on an inpatient setting.   Hospital wards have been, and continue to be, the situation that is most frequently used to teach the skills basic to the practice of medicine. When attending for a ward team, the teacher must address the needs of students with large differences in skill levels; some have only very basic concepts and abilities, while others have developed so they can both appreciate and learn the subtleties of medical practice.

Fortunately, learning medicine is a prolonged process. In fact, it should be a lifelong endeavor. Every student does not need to learn everything during this particular month. In most situations, the learners will return to the setting again during their training. Consideration of the level of the learner, the opportunities unique to the setting, and the medical procedures and facts that must be learned in a particular setting, enable the teacher to gain a necessary perspective and focus.

Inpatient settings generally provide an opportunity to teach skills in a less time-pressured situation than outpatient clinics. In clinics patients will be scheduled every twenty to thirty minutes, requiring residents to learn to manage brief encounters. Inpatient settings allow a more in-depth approach. Learners have an opportunity for continuous observation of patients that is not possible in an outpatient setting. This means that it is possible for students in this situation to learn much more about the evolution of a problem and the process of disease.

One of the disadvantages of the decreased length of the average hospital stay is that physicians-in-training do not have the same opportunity as in the past for intimate, close, observation of the natural history of diseases.

On an inpatient unit, residents and students have more frequent opportunities to talk with their patients, and, if they or a supervisor realize that an important piece of information or a physical finding has been missed, the patient is still there so that the omission can be remedied. They can observe the immediate effects of prescribed treatments and certainly have more control over whether or not their patients receive the treatment they have decided upon. The patient population is essentially "captive," a fact that must both be respected by the housestaff, but also used to promote learning. Unfortunately, students and residents usually fail to take advantage of this unique aspect of hospital care. Less than 10 percent of the time will a resident return to see a patient after morning rounds (Wray 1986).

During inpatient rotations, residents and students have a chance to work with other types of medical personnel, including nurses, respiratory therapists, physical therapists, pharmacists, and a host of other ancillary personnel.   All these people can serve as immediate resources for information and learning. Usually facilities are more centralized, so that diagnostic tests and procedures are more readily available, consultation results more immediately communicated, and the entire process of evaluation and treatment more efficient.

One of the increasingly complex aspects of medical care is communicating through the medical record. Certainly, ward rotations provide the opportunity for attendings to provide input to medical students and residents regarding the importance of documentation: what should and should not be included in a chart, and how to convey information clearly in written format.

In considering the roles of team members, the attending must cope with the wide range of abilities and level of skill among the various learners. Generally an inpatient service will consist of the attending, a supervisory or senior resident, a number of first year or junior residents of the attending's own specialty, and often residents of a different specialty. There are third year medical students, an occasional fourth year student, and maybe even a nurse practitioner student or two! Both the number of learners and their varied backgrounds can make the task of teaching seem overwhelming. If a team is well organized and both the attending and the supervisory resident are well prepared, teaching tasks can be shared. If each member of the team understands his role and what is expected, suddenly the burden of teaching can become much more reasonable.

Because medicine seems to be most easily taught case by case, emphasizing content, rather than process, it is easy to lose sight of the basic skills that students and residents must learn to become competent practitioners. Many attendings erroneously assume that all students and residents already possess these skills. Although some do, many will not, and almost everyone has room for improvement. For example, few would debate that the physician's most essential tool is the ability to take an accurate history and to perform a comprehensive physical examination. Yet, after completion of their physical diagnosis course, how frequently are students observed performing these important tasks?

When defining the roles of team members, the attending must initially assess the competency of each of the learners, starting with the supervisory resident. Is the supervisory resident competent? Can the resident accurately assess the clinical acumen of those he is supervising? Is the supervisory resident a good teacher, and can he relate effectively to the members of the ward team? The amount of the attending's direct involvement in both patient care and teaching is dependent upon the answers to these questions.

There are several methods for making this assessment. In many cases, the attending will have a prior opinion of the resident's clinical skills from working with him directly. Evaluations of the resident's previous work can be reviewed.   The most accurate method is to directly observe the resident during a clinical encounter. These same techniques can be applied to assessment of the resident's teaching skills.   Another very useful method is to ask the resident for a self-assessment, using the principle of "starting with the learner." Correlation of the resident's self-assessment with actual observation provides a basis for judging the accuracy of the resident's perception of himself and possibly of others.

During the process of evaluating the supervisory resident's skills, the attending can explain what he is doing and how he is doing it. In this way, the attending is modeling behaviors that the supervisory resident must learn.   One of the keys to learning how to be a good supervisor is learning to accurately assess the competency of subordinates. Just as the attending delegates responsibilities for clinical care and teaching to the supervisory resident, that resident must do so in turn to the first year residents and students.

Assessment of competency at the beginning of a rotation is essential not only for ensuring the quality of medical care, but also for tailoring teaching to the needs of the learners. This assessment is the first step in establishing an appropriate balance between the learner's knowledge and skills and the independence given.   The attending must individualize each learner's role in the delivery of care to meet his learning needs. In essence, those in supervisory roles must decide how much supervision is necessary. If the attending's assessment of the senior resident is that this resident has adequate clinical and teaching skills, the attending's role becomes much easier. The attending's role is to teach the senior resident how to be an effective supervisor. The attending can help the senior resident "fine tune" his patient management and teaching skills, add to the resident's knowledge base, and can share the task of teaching the junior residents and medical students. Acting as partners allows the attending and senior resident to divide the responsibities of teaching so that neither is overwhelmed.

The educational objectives for first year residents will be much less sophisticated. The direct responsibility for patient care may be new to some first year residents. Certainly the amount of independence granted to them should be more than what they have experienced as students. They will, therefore, need to learn additional skills and improve those they have already developed. First year residents should already have learned how to take a history and complete a physical examination when they were in medical school. They should have learned basic communication skills and should also possess some knowledge of differential diagnosis. During ward rotations, first year residents have an opportunity to upgrade their information gathering skills, including improving their history taking, their physical examination, and decisions regarding diagnostic testing.

New areas for learning include organizational skills, such as how to plan their day and how to use their time efficiently. They must now learn to prioritize, both their own time, and the urgency with which diagnostic and therapeutic procedures must be done for patients. They will need to increase their knowledge base and to develop patient management skills. They must both gain self-confidence and learn to recognize their own limits. They must develop communication skills with patients and with the health care team. This includes learning to present patients efficiently and effectively on rounds, as well as learning what needs to be included when writing concise notes in the chart. Most of these educational objectives can be met through the teaching of the supervisory resident.

Goals and objectives for third year medical students should be quite basic. They will need to learn how to take a history, how to do a physical examination, how to write an admission note, progress notes, and orders. They also need to learn something about the structure of the hospital setting: what roles each individual has, the process of admission and discharge, lines of communication, how to get help, and basic emergency procedures. These skills can be well taught by the first year residents.

This discussion is just an example demonstrating how the learning needs can be assessed and then divided among team members so that teaching can be more effective and efficient. Each setting will be unique, with different opportunities and different types of students.

Certainly, one of the ways to shorten the forty-day month is to take time to dissect the attending situation and organize the team so that responsibilities are shared.

CHAPTER 2

The Responsibilities of the Attending Physician

"The forty-day month" is certainly the way that the inpatient attending feels. For most academic physicians, "attending" is added on to other duties and obligations. For those who are actively involved in research, the laboratory essentially either shuts down, or the physician spends nights and weekends keeping things afloat. For the clinician, outpatient clinics must still be attended, patients seen and cared for. For everyone, no matter what academic position he holds, administrative tasks simply keep right on piling up. The added hours generally come from one place: one's personal life. In short, it's easy to be "burned out" on attending before the month even starts.

Despite these gruesome facts, attending in the hospital can be both exciting and fun. Most physicians became doctors because they wanted to take care of patients and were intrigued by the complexities of medicine. Hospitalized patients are usually the most in need of care and can be the most interesting and challenging cases. Seldom does a day go by without a new, puzzling, case being admitted. The fatigue and pressure of attending tend to be offset by the interest and excitement of the cases, the tremendous opportunity for teaching, if the attending is fortunate, and the enthusiasm of students and housestaff.

There are many different inpatient settings for which this book may be helpful. Although each setting is in its own way unique, the problems for attendings are quite similar. Whether teaching on a general inpatient ward or an intensive care unit, the process of teaching and learning is the same. The skills that students and residents need to learn in these settings will also be similar, but the stresses and the pace, for both students and teachers, will be different.

If academic physicians can develop skills related to this role, the task can become easier. Although it should seem obvious that preparing for a month of attending can be helpful in making that time more manageable, many physicians don't think much about it until the time has arrived. Some may not plan, believing that, because the patient load and the range of diseases that will be seen is unpredictable, there is no way to organize this time. Others may simply not want to consider the stresses and challenges until it is absolutely necessary. Whatever the reason, overcoming the inertia that can set in when thinking about the month can help you get a step ahead. Good preparation can reduce the stress of attending.

The beginning of good preparation cannot be done alone, but rather must be in conjunction with other physicians who share the same attending responsibilities. Generally, setting up meetings to discuss attending responsibilities would be the responsibility of the chief of service, the head of a division, or the residency program director. Special consideration could be given not only to discussion of the administrative details, such as assignment of rotations, but also to curriculum, teaching, and evaluation techniques.

One of the first issues to be addressed is the scheduling of attending rotations. It can be very helpful not only to discuss the time assigned to each attending, but also to define the optimal length of attending rotations for your specific setting. If a limited number of attendings are available to fulfill the assigned time, is it better to teach for a prolonged period of time infrequently, or for a shorter period more often? Typically, attending performance tends to decrease with the length of the rotation, with most doing less well with teaching and evaluation at the end of a rotation compared with the beginning.

For more demanding rotations, such as assignments for the intensive care unit, shorter rotations will be more conducive to sustained attending performance. The minimum length of rotations should be determined with consideration for continuity of care, resident and student evaluation, and for building a housestaff team.

Stress can be significantly reduced if each attending clears his schedule from as many other duties as possible. Consideration should be given to other personal and professional demands when assigning times. An attempt should be made to accommodate grant deadlines, annual meetings, and research presentations. Family matters, such as children's and spouse's vacation times, should be given equal weight.

One of the keys to good preparation is meeting with the resident who will be supervising the ward or intensive care unit team. If possible, at least two meetings should take place, one several months before the assigned rotation, and one shortly beforehand. During the first meeting, the resident and attending can coordinate residents' schedules, looking at continuity clinic assignments to adjust schedules so that there will always be adequate personnel available for coverage of the service. Although individual attendings are not generally responsible for assigning call schedules, both night and weekend call can be discussed, as well as mechanisms for covering sick days so that there is a mutual understanding of the expectations for the rotation. For example, expectations for resident reading and study will be quite different if call is assigned every fourth night compared with every third.

Times and frequency of attending rounds may also be discussed, as well as whether the attending will accompany the team during work rounds. Although the supervisory resident is obviously a subordinate, the attending should approach the resident in a collegial manner, modeling the behavior that is expected of the resident in his relationships with the students and interns. Thus, during the second meeting, the roles of the supervisory resident and the attending should be discussed and agreed upon.

One of the attending's major responsibilities is to teach the supervisory resident how to supervise. To do this, the attending must, on at least some occasions, observe the supervisory resident during work rounds, teaching medical students, and working with the junior residents. Methods and expectations for evaluation of the students and residents should be outlined. Regular meetings between the attending and the senior resident during the rotation are necessary both to review the supervisory resident's performance and how the clinical care and the teaching are being done. This second meeting is also a good time for the senior resident and attending to plan for the first day that the attending will be on-service.

It is wise to specifically plan time in advance of the attending rotation. Set aside enough time to complete the tasks that must be accomplished, considering which tasks must be done on a daily basis, which must be done weekly, and which at the end of the rotation. Assessing other activities that will be ongoing, mark the calendar so that tasks are given specific days and times. Scheduling regular meetings with the supervisory resident for a specified time each week will make these meetings much more likely to occur. This is particularly important in planning time for giving feedback to the residents and students on the service and evaluating them at the end. A portion of a day should be set aside at the middle and the end of the rotation for feedback and evaluation.

Some types of inpatient settings are conducive to preparation of a set curriculum. In intensive care units and on subspecialty services, it is highly likely that all residents will encounter specific problems, such as shock, malignant hypertension, or heart failure. On ward services, certain diseases are likely to occur with regularity during specific seasons. Even if patients with a particular problem are not admitted during a resident's rotation, there are core issues and approaches to problems that must be learned. Therefore, a curriculum can be considered and prepared. This is best done in conjunction with others who attend on the same unit, with the awareness that there are many curricular issues that will generate disagreement and discussion among attendings.

Differences in medical care between physicians can be quite dramatic. For example, there are as many approaches to the management of hypernatremic dehydration as there are attendings. In such instances, there is no single "right" way to manage the medical problem. If there were sufficient evidence to support a single method of care, that care would become "standard." Although these differences may not be medically significant, they have an important impact on the learning experiences of residents. The variance in practice can give residents a wonderful opportunity to observe different approaches to a problem and their relative effectiveness. On the other hand, these differences may also have a very negative impact on teaching situations. If attendings become quite rigid in both their own approach and their tolerance of varying methods of care, residents often find themselves caught between attendings in their arguments about correct medical care. These issues are ones that must be dealt with among physicians who share the responsibilities for attending on a unit.

Attending physicians should be aware of others' practices and be willing to discuss the pros and cons of each approach. This is not to say that unacceptable practices should be tolerated, or even that an attending must allow residents to use medical practices with which the attending is not comfortable. It is the attending physician who is ultimately responsible for the patient's care and the outcome. If, however, an attending is deviating from accepted standards of care and teaching residents and students also to do so, it is the responsibility of the committee for quality assurance and the chief of service to educate the attending.

Gathering articles and texts that are likely to be pertinent can be done in anticipation of the rotation. This time-consuming task can be shared with the supervisory resident, chief residents, other attendings, and with the medical librarian. In collecting materials it is important to remember the levels of the various learners who will be assigned to the service and the amount of time that each of the learners is likely to devote to reading. Gathering materials that are not likely to be read is a waste of time, effort, and money. Be realistic about the motivation for reading among the students, interns, and residents. Giving a single reading on a particular topic often is inappropriate. Students, particularly during their third year, have a relatively rudimentary understanding of most medical problems, whereas the knowledge of the supervisory resident should be more sophisticated.

Usually assignments from standard texts will be the most helpful for students. Good review articles (which unfortunately are often hard to find) are generally an excellent resource to use in teaching junior residents. Supervisory residents should appreciate the subtleties and variations of disease and disease presentation. They should be interested in the newest thoughts and research about various topics. Current literature from the journals will be appropriate to their learning.

Other literature that the supervisory resident may appreciate would be references that address teaching and managerial skills. Attending physicians should consider recommending materials which they found useful when they were residents. Two handbooks which may already be in your residency library are *Residents as Teachers: A Guide to Educational Practice* (Schwenk and Whitman 1984) and *The Chief Resident as Manager* (Whitman, Weiss, and Lutz 1988). To help hone our own managerial skills, attendings may wish to read *Executive Skills for Medical Faculty* (Whitman, Weiss, and Bishop (1989). These materials can be purchased from the Department of Family and Preventive Medicine, University of Utah School of Medicine, Salt Lake City, Utah 84132, Attention: Neal Whitman.

The main method that attendings use to carry out their teaching and patient care responsibilities is through rounds. Rounds have always been considered one of the primary methods for teaching students and residents how to practice medicine. In the opinion of Payson and Barchas, "Rounds are often the most important formal teaching exercise of clinical discipline... Rounds ... powerfully influence the orientation and performance of every new member of the profession" (1965). Yet, rounds are often very frustrating, dragging on for hours, without the attending or the resident achieving his purpose (Wilkerson *et al.* 1986).

The few studies of rounds that have been reported uniformly indicate that resident "work rounds" and attending "teaching rounds" are often suboptimal, both in terms of delivery of patient care and teaching (Payson 1961; Tremonti 1982; Wilkerson *et al.* 1986; Wray 1986). Work rounds are usually conducted by the senior resident without an attending present. They are focused on patient care and last approximately one hour.

In terms of delivery of patient care, work rounds are often deficient. Some portion of a physical examination is performed on approximately fifty percent of patients, but essential information, such as vital signs and medication sheets, are seldom reviewed. Approximately 25 percent of patients are not seen during work rounds, some because they are away from the ward for a procedure or test. Chronic patients are often bypassed. Work rounds account for most of the junior residents' contacts with their patients. Few return to see patients missed during rounds unless special procedures are performed or the patient's status changes acutely.

Examination of the teaching behaviors of the senior residents also reveals deficiencies in work rounds. Often the style of the supervisory resident is to take control, conducting interactions with patients, making the clinical decisions, and giving brief lectures. This style reduces the students and junior residents to a passive role. In only 11 percent of the encounters observed by Wilkerson *et al*. did the supervisory resident provide feedback on the clinical performance of team members (1986).

Faculty conduct teaching rounds in a distinctly different manner from resident rounds (Tremonti 1982). Faculty engage students and residents in problem-solving activities, a behavior that senior residents seldom employed. However, factors other than actual biomedical events were seldom discussed and never emphasized. Faculty spend much less time at the bedside than residents.

One of the problems is that rounds actually serve many different purposes. Those conducting rounds are generally expected to fulfil both a service commitment and an educational one. When a teacher is trying to meet multiple objectives simultaneously, the task becomes extremely difficult, if not impossible. An approach to this dilemma is to define the varied components of rounds, assess the learning opportunities, and limit the teaching objectives so they are congruent with the tasks being performed.

Each type of rounds will have a specific purpose and defined opportunities for learning. Although some types of rounding, such as work rounds and morning report, must be done daily, the frequency of other types of rounds should depend upon the skill levels of the residents and their learning needs. All too often, we expect far too much from our students, forgetting that adults are not able to incorporate large amounts of new knowledge at one time. A gradual approach with a logical progression is much more conducive to learning. Again, the teacher must balance the skills of the learner with responsibilities, so that there is enough stress to motivate the learner, but not so much that anxiety will interfere with learning.

Limiting objectives not only makes teaching more efficient and creative, it can make the task of attending less formidable, and may help attendings avoid "burn-out." Once the objectives of rounds have been decided, it is then easier to divide the teaching responsibilities among the members of the team. For example, the task on work rounds for the supervisory resident is to run rounds efficiently and to ensure that each member of the team understands what is expected of him for the remainder of the day. In order to accomplish this task, the supervisory resident must help students and junior residents learn how to make an effective and efficient presentation that includes a management plan. Thus, the the supervisory resident's teaching objective becomes congruent with the work that must be completed. Both during and after rounds, the senior resident has the opportunity to give immediate feedback regarding the presentations.

The following few paragraphs describe the function of different types of rounds. Options for the teaching setting for each type of rounds will also be described. Comfortable settings will improve the teaching atmosphere (unless some discomfort is necessary to keep people awake!)

Work rounds: Work rounds should be as short as possible. The team should round with a cart rack, with the head nurse, and with other key personnel who are responsible for the running of the ward. Presentations must be brief to avoid the discomfort of standing for long periods of time.

The purpose of work rounds is to inform the entire team of the patients who are being cared for by the team, to outline their problems, and to describe the work that must be accomplished during that day. At the end of rounds, each person involved should be knowledgeable enough about the patients so that, if the resident responsible for the primary care of that patient is absent from the ward, another can easily assume the responsibility for care. By the end of rounds, each student or resident must know what tasks must be accomplished during that day. They also should know with what urgency tasks must be completed. The supervisory resident must ascertain whether the students and residents understand how to accomplish their tasks (*e.g.* do they know what kind of MRI scan needs to be ordered and how to order it; do they know how to reach a specific consultant?). If they are unaware of the process the supervisor must assist them.

For the students and the junior residents, the learning experience should be how to make an efficient and effective presentation of new patients; how to logically, methodically, and concisely outline the patients' problems; how to briefly describe the most common diagnostic possibilities; and how to describe the management plan for the day, both in terms of diagnostic testing and therapeutic interventions. To be successful, the student must have examined the patient prior to work rounds, reviewed test results, and have read something about the patient's illness.

The educational experience for the supervising resident is to learn how to effectively guide the rounds, allowing the student or first year resident to reach his limits without letting him ramble or get too far off the track. Just as the attending needs to make the senior resident aware of his expectations, the senior residents should tell the students and junior residents what he expects. The senior resident should spend time with the students and junior residents to teach them how he wants to have patients presented. This can be done prior to the first time the senior resident actually makes rounds with the ward team. Work rounds then provide the supervisory resident with the opportunity to evaluate the students' and junior residents' presentation skills and to give immediate feedback. If the junior resident flounders with a presentation the supervisory resident could model the desired behavior.

The attending physician generally does not accompany the ward team on work rounds. Because work rounds provide the major opportunity for the senior resident to learn how to supervise, work rounds should be the responsibility of the senior resident. If, however, the attending does not occasionally accompany the team on work rounds, it is not possible for the attending to accurately assess the supervisory resident's teaching and managerial skills. When the attending is present for work rounds, his role is to quietly observe, unless there is an opportunity to model behaviors that the resident may not yet have. This should be discussed with the supervisory resident and should be done only with the permission of the resident. If approached in this manner the attendings presence does not undermine the position of the resident in his role as supervisor. It also models a very important behavior: respect for the resident as a person and a teacher. Generally it is wise to wait until after rounds to review the performance of the supervisory resident (see chapter eight, Assessment and Feedback).

Work rounds also provide an ideal opportunity for the attending to evaluate all the students and residents. During their presentations, it is likely that their thought processes will become obvious. Although this is not the time for demonstrating one's knowledge of esoterica, resident presentations will reveal the extent of their knowledge base and their awareness of how a problem might be approached. The teaching style of the supervisory resident is also readily observed. This will yield ample opportunity for the attending to interact with the senior resident about his communication skills, ability to give feedback, efficiency, and clarity in teaching.

Once the attending is satisfied that the supervisory resident is able to be effective in conducting work rounds, he should allow the resident increasing independence, attending work rounds only on occasions to monitor the progress of the supervisory resident and also that of the students and residents.

Morning report: The purpose of morning report is to inform the chief-of-service or the medical director of the hospital of the patients who are in the hospital. This allows the chief to know what medical and surgical

problems are being managed and gives him an opportunity to assess the quality of the medical care that is being
delivered. During morning report, the supervisory residents will also learn about the patients assigned to other
ward teams. The supervisory resident can then ask the
students and residents on his own service to see patients
who have unusual findings. This expands the experience
of the students and junior residents. Generally, morning
report should be given in a room that is large enough to
comfortably accommodate all those who need to be
present. A view box for x-rays and a blackboard are
desirable. Each attendee should be provided with a list
of patients admitted the night before and their diagnoses.
There should be enough room on the admit sheet for residents to take notes in the margins.

Morning report provides the chief with an opportunity to anticipate problems and to know how the medical and surgical services are functioning. It is another of
the quality assurance and risk management functions of a
hospital. It is also a time when problems with ancillary
services can be discovered and discussed with the residents who are providing the direct patient care. The
chief can learn about the function of the attendings who
are admitting patients to the hospital. If there are unusual occurrences, or repeated gaps in medical knowledge,
patient management, or teaching on the part of attendings, this should become obvious during morning report.

During morning report, senior residents present
patients and discuss differential diagnosis and patient

management. Just as work rounds provide the supervisory residents with the opportunity to teach presentation skills and problem solving, morning report is an important teaching situation for the chief-of-service. He can give immediate feedback to the supervisory residents on their presentations and on patient management.

Bedside Rounds: Bedside rounds should be done only on selected patients. It is not necessary for the attending to perform bedside rounds on the fiftieth baby who has been admitted for respiratory syncitial viral infection during an epidemic, unless the baby has an unusual or important finding. Bedside rounds are an opportunity for the attending or the supervisory resident to model behaviors for the students and junior residents. They can be used for the attending to take a history from the patient (a history that can be much more directed than the general history that the residents have taken and can fill in the gaps that the attending has determined in listening to the residents' presentations).

This is also a time when all students and residents can examine patients with abnormal physical findings. Again, this should be a very directed examination, including only those systems that have positive findings. This allows the attending to efficiently supervise each student's or resident's examination skills. Each should be required to repeat the examination until he has understood the finding. Although this may be intimidating to some residents, if it is done in an objective or collegial manner (*e.g.* "I always had difficulty hearing mid-systolic clicks when I was a resident, too"), the process can teach residents the importance of care, meticulousness, and the need for absolute honesty in the practice of medicine.

Bedside rounds also afford the opportunity for the attending to demonstrate communication skills. The attending can model behaviors that build rapport and enhance the doctor-patient relationship.

Attending Rounds: The purpose of attending rounds is to impart knowledge of a different kind. Attending rounds can be given in a comfortable, but cool, room that is well lit and preferably equipped with an x-ray view box, and, if possible, a microscope. This is the most appropriate place for the actual content of medicine and for problem-solving skills to be taught.

The attending's wider knowledge of each topic and his experience are important. All too often, attending rounds can become a competitive situation, with the practices of "one-upmanship" and the "guess what I'm thinking game" taking precedence over learning. Generally, attending rounds should take the form of a group discussion. However, flexibility in the format of rounds is important. If the disease being discussed is one that is relatively rare, it may be much more appropriate for the attending to give a short lecture and assign readings on the topic.

At the next session, it is then wise to review what the residents were supposed to learn. This can sometimes be very surprising. If attendings learn to review the last session, they will rapidly have ample evidence that adult learners usually remember only a few important facts. They will much more readily remember situations. The more familiar the context of the learning experience, the more that they will then be able to "fit in" the pieces. Thus rather than listing facts and differential diagnosis, a better teaching technique would be to assign the task of briefly reviewing the topic presented to one of the students or residents. This is one way of slightly increasing tension, making the motivation for the learner a bit greater. Attending rounds provide one of the best settings for the students and residents to learn problem solving skills.

In the first chapter, we discussed the role of attending physicians in terms of balancing the medical needs of patients admitted to their ward and the educational needs of medical students and residents assigned to work under their supervision. In this chapter, we addressed the responsibilities of attending physicians in terms of work rounds, morning report, bedside rounds, and attending rounds. In the next chapter, we will identify the types of learning that attending physicians should help medical students and residents achieve in these settings.

Chapter 3

The Objectives of Learning

Teaching knowledge is important. This knowledge can be viewed as levels of *cognition*. In the taxonomy developed by Bloom and colleagues (1956), the lowest level of cognition concerns facts. Are there facts students did not know before their rotation on your service that they now know? We could expect so. At a higher level of cognition, we also would expect students to be able to extrapolate and interpret some of these facts. In other words, there is now comprehension that was not there before. In addition, they should be able to apply this knowledge when they see future patients. There is application from one situation to another.

There are higher levels of cognition which may or may not be beyond the scope of a medical student, but definitely are within the range of a resident: analysis (ability to organize principles and establish relationships), synthesis (ability to develop models and identify patterns) and evaluation (ability to make judgments).

In addition to learning knowledge, medical students and residents are expected to learn new skills. This domain of learning, known as *psychomotor*, concerns medical procedures which will be addressed in chapter six. But, when asked what they want students and residents to learn on their clinical service, many physicians recognize that there is more than knowledge and skills.

This recognition was shared by Dr. Lloyd Smith who identified his purposes and priorities in teaching as, "First, to inspire. Second, to challenge. Third, and only third, to impart information" (1984, p. 6). Inspiration and challenge address a third domain of learning. In addition to knowledge and skills, ward attendings also are concerned with teaching about attitudes, beliefs, and values. This is known as the *affective* domain of learning.

Affective learning is not isolated from cognitive and psychomotor learning. With regard to cognitive learning, medical students and residents will...

• *acquire new knowledge only if they want to receive it;*

• *comprehend it only if they are willing to understand it;*

• *apply the information only if they value it;*

• *analyze and synthesize it only if they internalize it;*

• evaluate it only if they see how it fits into their medical practice.

With regard to psychomotor learning, medical students and residents will learn a new skill if they feel...

• comfortable doing it;

• confident in themselves; and

• responsible for its accomplishment.

The integration of all domains of learning occurs in the process of medical problem solving. As described by Kassirer and Kopelman (1991), at the start of a diagnostic encounter, physicians generate hypotheses from a set of findings and use those hypotheses to guide data collection. These diagnostic hypotheses form a context in which further information gathering takes place. As new findings emerge, a working hypothesis is formulated that is used to further action. Obviously, the diagnostic approaches used are limited by the physician's domain of knowledge and his data collection skills. But, in addition, attitude plays a key role in the process of generating and verifying diagnostic hypotheses. In the field of chemical engineering, Woods (1983) identified ten such attitudes which Whitman and Schwenk (1991) believe are relevant to medical problem solving and should be promoted by clinical teachers:

1. Are we careful?

2. Are we attentive?

3. Are we curious?

4. Are we skeptical

5. Are we honest?

6. Are we objective?

7. Are we receptive to new ideas?

8. Are we systematic?

9. Are we decisive?

10. Are we persistent?

In the relationship between affective learning and cognitive and psychomotor learning, we can view affective learning as means to the ends. In other words, the learner's attitudes, beliefs, and values may be necessary for cognitive and psychomotor learning to be possible. In supervising medical students and residents, you probably have observed that for meaningful learning to occur, there must be a transformation and evaluation of the information so that it can be used in the future. John Dewey pioneered this concept when he said that,

Learning is problem-solving in which the person continually evaluates his experience in the light of its foreseen and unforeseen consequence...learning is not simply acquisition, but a moment of experience out of which emerges redefined purposes, new evaluations, and action in the sense of continued growth (Ratner 1939).

Emotions play a key role in learning. Essentially, we remember what we understand, we understand what we pay attention to, and we pay attention to what we want to. That is why John Russell, the art critic of the *New York Times* commented, "No two human beings read the same book, watch the same movie, hear the same music or look at the same paintings and sculpture. Different eyes and different ears are at work, and different expectations." Similarly, we could say that no two physicians examine the same patient!

In addition to its role as a means to an end, affective learning can, itself, be an end. Are there attitudes, beliefs, and values regarding the medical profession and the care of the patient which you would like medical students and residents to share with you? If so, how do you teach these? Will a lecture (sermon) do it? Not likely. Instead, in working with medical students and residents, there is a process of establishing "professional intimacy" acting as a "role model" and "mentor," and engaging them in the "conversation of medicine." Each of these terms will be addressed with the aim of helping attending physicians develop their own style and approach to teaching attitudes, beliefs, and values.

PROFESSIONAL INTIMACY

Medical student and resident performance will be enhanced when their teachers are emotionally close without being necessarily personal friends– a delicately balanced relationship called "professional intimacy" (Whitman and Schwenk 1984). An analogous relationship exists between doctors and patients. On one hand, it is neither possible nor desirable for physicians to make every patient a close, personal friend. On the other hand, it is helpful for physicians to not hide behind a facade.

Being professionally intimate with medical students and residents means *sharing your thoughts and values* in a manner that encourages them to share theirs with you and *demonstrating comfort* with learners of different abilities and backgrounds. Faculty who are professionally intimate often become positive "role models" for medical students and residents, *i.e.*, someone who does not *tell* others how to be but can *show* them and, by example, make being that way seem desirable and worthwhile.

When teachers are professionally intimate, the "psychological distance" between teachers and learners lessens so that it becomes possible for medical students, residents, and faculty to teach each other and to engage in a "conversation of medicine" in which all participants become learners.

ROLE MODELS

Role modeling, or teaching by example, is intrinsic to the process of teaching. Medical teachers are, whether they realize it or not, role models for medical students and residents. Basic science teachers serve as role models by demonstrating the scientific method, including hypothesis testing. Clinical teachers serve as role models by demonstrating medical problem-solving and bedside manners. Both basic science and clinical teachers role model by conveying enthusiasm for their work.

Teachers identified by graduating medical students as enthusiastic were enlisted by the University of Chicago Pritzker School of Medicine to interview patients in front of a class of second-year medical students and, afterwards, to discuss these interviews with the students. Siegler *et al.* (1977) reported that, based on student questionnaires, this simple change in the curriculum had a positive effect on student attitudes and that "the use of such role models should be considered as a means of improving the teaching of the doctor-patient relationship and of improving students' attitudes about the importance of interpersonal skills" (p. 937).

In order to promote role modeling, the Indiana University School of Medicine convened a conference for approximately 100 faculty members, community physicians, residents, and medical students, at which they concluded that role modeling was essential to instilling within students the desire to become lifelong learners (Ficklin *et al.* 1988).

Of course, although the Indiana participants identified both positive and negative aspects of role modeling, when some educators use the term, "role model," they assume a positive influence. However, role models can be positive or negative. In order to become a positive role model, medical teachers should consider four areas of professional behavior (Whitman and Schwenk 1984).

1. *Be capable.* You can teach medical students and residents to become competent clinicians by providing excellent medical care, being organized in your patient care and your teaching, being well-read in your field, and demonstrating how you value the development of your own abilities.

2. *Be sensitive.* You can teach medical students and residents to be sensitive by your being sensitive to them as well as to your patients. By being empathic to the anxieties of being a medical learner, being patient with their efforts to learn, and being compassionate about their failures and gentle in recognizing their inadequacies, in other words, by treating your students and residents as you would like them to treat their patients, you will encourage proper approaches to patient care.

3. *Be enthusiastic.*   By showing interest in patients, medical students and residents become interested, as well. In addition, by being accessible to medical students and residents, interested in their problems and needs, and energetic in your approach to them, you will promote productive learning as well as good patient care. Most studies of teaching identify the importance of enthusiasm.

4. *Be yourself.*   There is no single "good" personality type in Medicine. But, all positive role models are honest about how they deal with the uncertainties, difficulties, and ambiguities of medical practice.

In addition to considering these four areas of professional behavior, Irby (1986) suggests that to be an *intentional* role model, medical teachers should articulate the mental processes that led to the successful completion of a diagnosis or clinical procedure. By demonstrating a skill *and* labelling its important aspects, students and residents will be better enabled to imitate it.

By being professionally intimate with all medical students and residents, a medical teacher will become a role model for some. By being a role model for some medical students and residents, a medical teacher may become a "mentor" for a few.

MENTORS

Ward attendings should consider becoming a mentor to *one or two* learners. Not all teachers become mentors, and not all medical students or residents have one. In considering the mentor's role, we recognize that the relationship between a mentor and his protege is the ultimate teacher-student interaction.

The literature on mentoring is almost exclusively written in the male gender because traditionally women have had few mentors, male or female, and female mentors are scarce. As more women enter medical school, and ultimately become medical school faculty, this is changing. As described in the male tradition, Levinson (1978) identified several functions of the mentor which should be considered for men and women entering the field of medicine:

> He may act as a teacher to enhance the young man's skills and intellectual development. Serving as sponsor, he may use his influence to facilitate the young man's entry and advancement. He may be a host and guide, welcoming the initiate into a new occupational and social world and acquainting him with its values, customs, resources, and cast of characters. Through his own virtues, achievements, and way of living, the mentor may be an exemplar that the protege can admire and

seek to emulate. He may provide counsel and moral support in time of stress. The mentor has another critical function... developmentally the most critical one: to support and facilitate the realization of the Dream (p. 98).

Dr. R. William Betcher is a psychiatrist who was a clinical psychologist before entering medical school. As a medical student at Harvard Medical School he wrote *A Student Guide to Medical School: Study Strategies, Mneumonics, Personal Growth* (1985). In this helpful book, he recommends medical students stay in touch with their dream of being a doctor and try to reconcile their life structure to the dream, not the other way around. Mentors can play a key role in helping medical students by believing in them and in their dreams.

The University of Wisconsin Medical School has expanded the notion of one-to-one mentoring with a class mentor program which provides a senior physician mentor to an entire class of students throughout its four years in medical school. One of their objectives was to use the experience of a senior clinician to help students realize how the information and concepts they learn are important to the practice of Medicine (Lobeck and Stone 1990). While one physician cannot become a personal mentor to each student, a potential benefit could be to alert the students to the need for mentoring which could occur when they work with ward attendings in the third and fourth years of medical school.

In adopting the role of mentor, ward attendings should consider that they, as well as the protege, can benefit from the relationship. For mentors, this relationship may meet their need to create and care for new life! Moreover, in the very act of guiding and promoting others, mentors act to effect their own growth and development (Healy and Welchert 1990).

THE CONVERSATION OF MEDICINE

Dr. Lewis Thomas observed that science is taught as if its facts were somehow superior to the facts in other scholarly disciplines, although, in reality, every field of science is incomplete (1982). The same could be said of medicine. The uncertainties of medicine were highlighted by Bursztajn *et al.* who described a "probabilistic paradigm" in their thoughtful book, *Medical Choice, Medical Chances* (1981). Medical teachers should consider that there may not be a universal structure behind "knowledge," but rather a temporary consensus arrived at by the medical community. If we are really concerned with training physicians for the twenty-first century, perhaps medical schools will be most effective when their students actively participate in the continuous conversation that occurs in medicine (Bruffee 1984).

There is a myth of medical education that students have to learn the vocabulary of medicine before they begin to participate in its discussion. For medical students to be able to participate in the conversation of medicine, it is important that they learn a vocabulary, of course, but not a dictionary (Bishop 1984) *and this vocabulary can be learned in the process of medical problem solving.* As described by one faculty developer,

> Good teaching will help more and more people learn to speak and listen in the community of truth, to understand that truth is not in the conclusions so much as in the process of conversation itself, that if you want to be "in truth" you must be in the conversation (Palmer 1990, p. 12).

One metaphor we find helpful is to compare a school to a cocktail party. A newcomer enters a room where various conversations are occurring in clusters. When the newcomer walks up to a small group, he first must listen to find out what the conversation is about. Soon, he feels ready to contribute to the dialogue. At some point, a few people leave the group for another and others arrive. Eventually, our "newcomer" joins another cluster, as well. The medical school is one cocktail party where the conversation of medicine occurs in various courses and clinical rotations. But, this conversation also goes on elsewhere, wherever medicine is practiced. Perhaps this is why Dr. Lloyd Smith warned us that one of the dangers of current medical education is it leads to graduation from medical school. In his view, "The true physician never graduates from medical school; he simply transfers" (Smith 1985).

In this chapter, we identified three domains of learning: cognitive, psychomotor, and affective. The reader's own personal experience probably confirms the finding that medical knowledge, skills, and attitudes are learned in an integrative fashion. Nowhere is this more obvious that in the learning of communication skills. How to teach communication skills is the subject of the next chapter.

CHAPTER 4

Teaching Communication Skills

The world of physicians and medical students in teaching hospitals is, to a great extent, like all worlds, defined, expressed, and limited by its language, a language that illuminates disease and technology but consigns to shadow much of the uniquely human in patient and doctor... I believe that there is a major, insufficiently appreciated reason for the sorry state of medicine's language for and about the subject of its activities, the human being: the unexamined assumption that the scientific way of knowing is the only way of knowing anything germane to the doctor's tasks. (William J. Donnelly 1986).

The art of communication is one of the most important aspects of clinical medicine. No matter what specialty a physician practices, he must be able to communicate effectively with others, both verbally and through writing. Residents and students must learn to have effective interchanges not only with patients and their families, but also with other physicians, nurses, social workers, ward clerks, laboratories, and a myriad of others. Although in recent years, medical schools and residency programs have begun to emphasize and teach medical interviewing skills (Lipkin 1984; Quirk 1986; Lichstein 1985), little attention has been paid to other types of communication, such as writing and communication with peers and hospital staff (Yanoff 1988). Ward rotations offer unique learning opportunities to medical learners, particularly with regard to peer interactions, interactions with a medical team, and in learning to create an accurate, complete, medical record. The purpose of this and the next chapter is to assist ward attendings in their role in teaching students skills that are critical to their eventual success as physicians.

CASE PRESENTATIONS ON ROUNDS

The Random House Dictionary defines communication as the imparting or interchange of thoughts, opinions, or information by speech, writing, or signs. During ward rotations, communication with peers is usually done during work rounds, attending rounds, and the one-to-one exchanges between the supervisory resident, the attending, and the students and residents. The structure of work rounds was discussed in chapters one and two in which the need for balancing the conflict between the needs for patient care and teaching were emphasized. Likewise, there are conflicts that must be resolved in giving case presentations. Attendings and the supervisory resident must help students and junior residents resolve the conflict between the need for efficient, concise, objective presentations, and the need for all members of the ward team to be aware of the patient as a person.

Poirier, in a provocative discussion of the language of medical discourse, asks, "Is the story being told in the medical report the story of the patient's life or of the physician's relationship with the patient's illness" (1988)? She points out that the case report, by its very nature, is a purposeful, carefully ordered communication, that then can create the danger of depersonalizing the patient. Students need to learn to resolve this tension with the help of attendings, so that their presentations are not so businesslike that the patient is forgotten. They must also become aware that "*objective*" is not synonymous with "*impersonal*." This can be done by insisting that an appropriate amount of social information be included in the presentation. This not only can give the listeners a picture of the patient as a human being, but is necessary because psychosocial factors are critical to the management of the patient and his illness.

Another method is to insist that presenters speak in the first person. Use of the passive voice allows the speaker to avoid direct references to him or herself in relationship to the patient. Poirier states it succinctly: "A written and oral style that does not use 'I' or active verb forms with which to discuss a patient discourages a sense of medicine as a personal, active, and interactive enterprise." Use of passive verbs and the third person, as is so commonly seen not only in presentations, but also in journal articles and other types of medical communications, also allows the student or resident to avoid taking direct responsibility for his actions. Saying "A lumbar puncture was done, and an EEG was ordered" is quite different than reporting, "I did a lumbar puncture and then ordered an EEG."

Schwenk and Whitman (1987), in their discussion of the use of an efficient logistical format for case presentations, outline the traditional case presentation. Residents and students should use the well-known SOAP format developed by Weed (1968). The presentation of new patients should include the chief complaint, history of present illness, past medical history, social history, review of systems, tests ordered and their results, assessment of problem, treatment and outcome. On work rounds, the emphasis should be on the present illness, with the past medical history and review of systems being quite focused, so that only very pertinent positive and negative information is included. Psychosocial information, as discussed above, should also be included. In this manner, even the most complicated patients can be presented in no more than five minutes. Efficiency is needed not only so that rounds can be completed in a timely manner, but also because the average listener cannot retain all the facts beyond a seven minute presentation (Yurchak).

Presentation of patients after the initial hospital day can be more brief. It seems superfluous to say that all patients should be reviewed during work rounds, but as discussed in chapter two, as many as one quarter of the patients may not be seen during rounds (Wray 1986).

Students and junior residents should evaluate patients daily, including review of the nurses notes, the patient's vital sign sheet, review of all medications and treatments and the patient's reaction, examination of all laboratory data. They should make an assessment of the patient's physical and emotional status, performing pertinent portions of the physical examination. They should discuss with the patient how he is feeling, the results of tests, and management plans for the day. This all-important aspect of medical care is frequently overlooked.

The student will then be adequately prepared to present the patient on rounds. This includes a discussion of the patient's current medical condition, any pertinent, new historical information, the results of tests, procedures, and consultation, an assessment of the patient, and the management plan. The management plan should include a list of current treatments and medications, the patient's response, and plans for both diagnostic tests and proposed changes in treatments.

As physicians progress through their medical training, they learn to become more efficient in their case presentations. This can be one of the more difficult skills for medical students to learn. They are frequently "on the spot" during work and attending rounds, having to expose their ignorance and lack of skill in oral presentation. It is advisable for the supervisory resident to have both group and individual teaching sessions with those he supervises to work on presentation skills early in the rotation.

During teaching rounds, the form of presentation will be somewhat different than on work rounds. The objectives of work rounds are to present patients efficiently, concisely, and to devise a management plan for the day. The purpose of teaching rounds is to help students and residents learn clinical problems solving. If fewer, more detailed presentations are made, using the same format as outlined above, time will be available for the attending to use an inquiry mode. Clinical teachers can ensure that their interactions stimulate problem-solving by asking questions that are open-ended and divergent.

One technique to use during case presentations is to try to emulate the process of problem-solving that physicians use in practice: early hypothesis formation with subsequent testing information against those hypotheses. After presenting the chief complaint, the student or resident is asked to name *the most common* conditions that produce the symptom complex. He then relates the history of present illness. At the conclusion of this, the attending may ask both the presenter and the group what information supports the various possible diagnoses, whether more specific history would be helpful in differentiating the diseases, and whether the information suggests other possibilities than those originally given.

After presentation of the past medical history, the teacher asks the group how the past condition of the patient could affect the proposed diagnoses, *e.g.* does the chronic condition make certain diagnoses more or less likely, does it suggest another etiology for the symptoms, or change the presentation of the illness? Questions can also be asked in an anticipatory manner: "If indeed this were a tubal pregnancy rather than appendicitis, what might you find on physical examination?"

This approach emphasizes the importance of pertinent negatives, as well as pertinent positive findings, when the presenter is asked to detail the examination. Asking questions regarding what laboratory findings would either support or contradict each condition prior to the resident's presenting laboratory data will also teach medical learners to be more specific in their reasoning for ordering tests and may help with synthesis of the information when it is available.

Although this process may seem tedious, and does not allow display of esoterica, it emphasizes the process of thinking, using the medical content to support diagnostic reasoning. The most common errors in diagnostic reasoning are: 1) *omission,* in which an important clinical clue is simply ignored; 2) *premature closure,* when the diagnosis of the patient's condition is less than justified by existing data; or 3) *wrong synthesis*, in which the available data contradict the conclusions (Voytovich). Generally, by the end of such a discussion, a logical, efficient, diagnostic and therapeutic plan can be devised. Often, with careful history taking, a good physical examination, and a few laboratory tests, there will be enough information to make a firm diagnosis or narrow the possibilities to just a few entities.

This is just one method of using the inquiry mode. Schwenk and Whitman, in their book *The Physician as Teacher*, provide a discussion of teaching rounds, and using questions to promote problem-solving. They list some specific types of questions that can be asked during each portion of the presentation. These questions are designed to help students "clarify, support, defend, justify, correlate, critique, evaluate, analyze, interpret, and predict..." rather than to "regurgitate facts or answers with one or a few words."

COMMUNICATION WITH ATTENDINGS

Students and housestaff need to be made aware of the necessity for consistent communication with the physician of record (the patient's attending physician). If the hospital attending is not the patient's primary care physician, it is imperative that some method of continuing intercourse with the primary physician also be developed. Expectations for communication should be clearly delineated at the beginning of each student's or resident's rotation. Lines of communication should be explained, so that students know both how to contact the attending and when they are expected to do so. Thus, the supervisory resident should have the attending's pager number, office number, and home telephone number. If the attending anticipates being unavailable for a period of time, the supervisory resident will need to know whom he should call in the attending's absence. The reverse is also true: the attending should be able to contact the supervisory resident easily, so he must know the resident's pager number, home telephone number, and whom to contact when the resident is not on the ward (*e.g.* for continuity clinic).

Often students and residents are not aware of the ethical and legal issues regarding confidentiality. They are frequently unconscious of the fact that they must be careful about when, where, and with whom they discuss their patients. More than once, lawsuits have resulted from conversations that were overheard as physicians were talking about patients in the hospital elevator or the cafeteria! They may receive calls from friends, relatives, and strangers requesting information about their patients. This issue is particularly difficult in pediatrics when parents are separated or when grandparents call. Remind the students and residents that information can only be shared with the physicians of record, the patient (or parent in the case of minors), and others to whom the patient voluntarily releases information.

Communication with the attending of record

The attending should be readily available for consultation when the housestaff need help with a patient. He should also clearly state under what circumstances he wishes to be contacted for the patients for whom he is directly responsible.

This generally would include: 1) notification at the time of admission of new patients; 2) a telephone conversation regarding the new patient's condition and management, after the housestaff has evaluated the patient; 3) immediate notification of any significant change in the patient's condition; 4) notification and discussion of recommendations made by consultants prior to implementation of those recommendations; and 5) notification of significant changes in the management plan that are made *after* morning rounds.

The extent to which attendings need to maintain contact with the students and residents will vary with the capabilities of the residents and the style of the attending. Once "ground rules" have been established, they should be maintained. Any deviation from the system that is established should be discussed with the housestaff.

Communication with the patient's primary care physician

This is a neglected area of communication that can cause many conflicts between physicians. It is probably the primary source of the "town/gown" separation between the community of practicing physicians and those at the medical center. Good communication between these two groups can do nothing except improve patient care, education, and the exchange of information. Even if the primary care physician does not want to be directly involved with the patient's hospitalization, he will often have a great deal of information that can be useful in the patient's management. This will be particularly true at the time of a patient's admission when the primary care physician can give the students and residents an assessment of such factors as past medical conditions that may affect the patient's course, the patient's compliance with prescribed treatments, and pertinent psychosocial information.

At the time of discharge, the primary care physician will not only need information regarding follow-up plans, but also may assist in discharge planning because he will know about the family's situation. It is not necessary to have the students and residents responsible for all contacts with the primary physician. That expectation will guarantee failure of the system! Certainly, at the time of admission, the primary care physician should be contacted. At that time, the resident or student can ascertain needed information, and can also inquire whether or not the primary physician wants to be directly involved with the patient's care during the hospitalization.

During the patient's hospital stay, the residents may request that the patient's primary nurse call the physician's office with a daily report. The nurse can talk with the physician's office nurse. Not only is this good for public relations, most nurses will then feel more involved in the patient's care. They often will get useful information from the primary physician's staff. At the time of discharge, the student or resident can ask the discharge planner to contact the primary physician's office to invite a representative to come to the discharge planning meeting if there is one. At a minimum, the primary care doctor needs to know: 1) When the patient is discharged; 2) The discharge diagnoses; 3) What medications that the patient is taking, the exact dosage, and any expected side effects from medications; 4) What plans for follow-up have been made, *e.g.* if and when the patient is to see a specialist. Timely dictation and transmission of discharge summaries to the primary physician is essential.

COMMUNICATING WITH ALLIED HEALTH
PERSONNEL

After the initial hospital day, students and residents spend an average of less than ten minutes a day with the ward patients for whom they are caring (Wray 1986). The care of these patients must be coordinated, and it is the physician who is responsible for ensuring that this occurs. Effective communication between the members of the medical team are crucial. Poor or inaccurate communication can not only lead to inefficiency and prolongation of the hospital stay, but may be the source of errors. Communication problems are also frequently mentioned as an important source of job dissatisfaction among non-physician health care providers (Farley 1989).

Studies of communication systems within organizations have indicated that there are several important factors that lead to effective interchanges among employers and employees. These include a positive communicate atmosphere, direct and clear lines of communication between employees and their immediate superiors, and personal feedback on job performance (Pincus 1986). Organizations develop "rules" for communication. Some of these rules are very standardized and formal, such as communication through the medical record. Others are more informal. Essentially, the rules, whether clearly defined or unspoken, define what behavior is required, what is preferred, and what is prohibited in a certain context (Farley 1989).

Within the context of the ward team, there is certainly a hierarchy of personnel and both explicit and implicit rules for communication with staff. In their communications with staff, students and residents need to have attitudes that will facilitate positive interactions. Key among these is treating others with respect, and learning the skill of active listening.

Observing the medical learner's interactions with other health professionals will give the attending information about the learner's self-concept. Those who are insecure are much more likely to have difficulty listening to those they consider to be below them in the hierarchy. They may treat their "inferiors" in a dictatorial manner, rather than eliciting cooperation. This style will only stifle the exchange of information and can be very detrimental to the care of patients.

Effective communication between housestaff and others will have certain characteristics. First among them is clear communication channels. These channels are links among all those responsible for the patient's care. In order for these channels to be open, there must be a leader responsible for coordination of the patient's care who is readily available (the student, resident, or attending), defined roles for each member of the team (who is responsible for what, *e.g.* the nurse will call the primary care physician's office today), respect, cooperation, and trust among those who are responsible, and accepted methods of both written and verbal communications. Using the principles of feedback discussed in chapter eight, residents can learn ways of resolving conflicts when disagreements arise regarding either the roles and responsibilities of the staff or the management of patients.

The importance of clarity of messages cannot be overemphasized. Problems with clarity with verbal messages can occur when there are multiple definitions for the same word, when personal interpretations of words differ, and when dual messages are given. This can be particularly true in the field of medicine in which the use of jargon is rampant. Often, the listener will not ask for clarification, because he will be embarrassed and assume that he is supposed to know what was meant. One method for avoiding errors in verbal interactions is for the resident to ask the listener to repeat what he heard. In this manner, both the listener and the speaker can know at the end of the conversation that their idea of what should be done is congruent.

Clarity of written messages is most frequently threatened by the illegibility of the residents' and students' handwriting. This, and another problem, simply failing to record information, are discussed in chapter five.

COMMUNICATING WITH PATIENTS

One of the most fundamental characteristics necessary for the practice of medicine is the intelligent, sensitive, and systematic collection of information from patients. The medical history is the doctor's most valuable tool (Hampton 1975). In order for medical learners to become competent in this process, they must be systematically taught and encouraged to continually improve. Interestingly, excellent interviewers spend no more time with patients than those who are less skilled, but they are able to elicit more information from patients (Platt 1979; Carter 1982). Even the most skilled interviewers will comment that the process of learning how to elicit, understand, and integrate information during a patient encounter requires constant refinement. Thus, even the supervisory resident will have many skills that can be improved.

Teaching doctor-patient communication is difficult and time-consuming. Although effective communication between doctor and patient should be one of the objectives of ward rounds, van der Merwe found that of 10 department heads who responded to a questionnaire, only one listed communication as an objective for his rounds (1989). The task of teaching doctor-patient communications can seem overwhelming to a ward attending; however, it can be done (Maguire). The first important step is to be a good role model. An attending's demonstration of care and concern for the patients' welfare is paramount. When seeing patients on rounds, the attending can demonstrate effective communication skills, starting with using the patient's name, speaking in a friendly tone of voice, listening to the patient, and being sensitive to non-verbal cues. In reality, the first time to demonstrate these skills is in working with the ward team! On the first day, the attending can introduce himself, learn the names of each member of the ward team, speak with a friendly, non-intimidating tone of voice, listen to the team members, and finally, be aware of their non-verbal cues.

In order to assess the extent to which he must teach interviewing skills, the ward attending should know something about the curriculum of the medical school and the residency program. Because there is insufficient time during ward rotations to teach basic interviewing skills, this should not be the responsibility of the ward attending. Medical students should already have had a course on the medical interview. Residents should also have opportunities during their postgraduate education to learn interviewing techniques in a structured setting.

The attending has the opportunity to add to basic skills through observation of the students and residents. He can teach skills through role-modeling. It is the attending's responsibility, however, to make an assessment of this most basic and important skill. Additionally, as indicated by the study of Romm *et al.*, physicians are particularly poor in their communications with patients regarding discussion of the diagnosis, tests, and treatment plans. The attending should stress these points with the students and residents and attempt to help them improve through role-modeling, observation, and feedback regarding their interactions. Table 4.1 outlines the attending role in teaching residents and students doctor-patient communications.

Just as important as skills are the attitudes of the medical learners. In order to establish rapport with a patient, physicians must learn to have unconditional positive regard for patients, to respect them and their values. They must be able to approach patients in a nonjudgmental manner. This can be extremely difficult, particularly when the values of the physician and the patient are very divergent. Other attitudes that need to be developed include respect for the patient's individuality and autonomy, enlistment of the patient as a partner, and a willingness to learn from others.

Attending physicians are accomplished interviewers, and as such, are often "unconsciously competent." They have been able to do what they do so well for so long, that they are no longer aware of the process or the specific skills that they possess. Attendings must make an effort to be more aware of what the components of a medical interview are and how they use them. Table 4.2 is adapted from an article by Lipkin *et al.* that describes a core curriculum for residencies in internal medicine on the medical interview. The table lists examples of basic skills.

CONGRUENT TEACHING

We read in the *Wall Street Journal* that money-back guarantees, usually limited to such items as tarnished toasters or cold pizza, have found a new home: academia (March 19, 1991). It was reported that a professor at a business school decided to practice what he preaches (teaches) by offering a money-back guarantee to graduate students taking his course on the management of service operations. If they are not satisfied with the way he has taught, he will pay them $250.00 toward class fees, all out of his own pocket!

This professor explained that his intent was to bring the real world to what he teaches in the course, which examines case studies of top-notch service companies such as Dominos Pizza and Federal Express. While we are not recommending that attending physicians pay medical students and residents who are dissatisfied with the teaching, we are suggesting that they make how they teach congruent with what they teach. In other words, just as this business professor tries to make how he teaches consistent with what he teaches (in his case, the delivery of quality service), attending physicians should make how they communicate with medical students and residents consistent with the what they teach (in their case, the delivery of quality care).

The principle of congruence comes to mind when a course on patient interviewing begins with asking medical student to introduce themselves to each other and to state what are their expectations. This opening could mirror the patient interview process which begins with the introductions and the patient's chief complaint. The principle also is evident when a seminar on medical ethics begins with asking residents what groundrules they think would facilitate discussion. Perhaps to encourage open discussion, the residents might suggest that all comments made in the seminar be considered confidential. Can you see how this discussion of seminar groundrules could anticipate the ethical dimensions of confidentiality?

Likewise, we view the communication skills used by the attending physician with medical students and residents, both verbal and written, as an opportunity to demonstrate the communication skills he wishes them to use with him, each other, allied health personnel, and patients. Similarly, in approaching the "learning" problems of the medical students and residents, could the attending model the same hypothetico-deductive approach used in approaching the diagnosis of a patient's problem?

We strongly urge attending physicians to use their creativity to make how they teach congruent with what they teach. Of course, it would be understandable if the reader thinks an economics professor went too far when he offered students in his course on consumerism an opportunity to buy their grades!

In this chapter, we suggested how to teach communication skills in an integrative fashion. In the teaching of communication skills, it is obvious that attending physicians cannot separate knowledge, attitude, and skills. In fact, this integration also occurs in the teaching of medical procedures, the subject of chapter six. But first let's extend our discussion of communication skills with a brief review of a special kind of communication, the medical record.

Table 4.1 Attending role in teaching doctor-patient communications

1. Role-modeling to assist learners in improving their skills.

2. Observation of student and resident interactions with patients so that an adequate evaluation of the skills can be made.

3. Emphasis and teaching of skills that have been shown to be deficient in most physicians, specifically daily communication with patients regarding the diagnosis, tests to be done, the result of completed tests, and treatment plans.

Table 4.2 Examples of skills necessary for good interviewing technique

Competently elicit the patient's story of illness that includes a detailed delineation of symptoms while at the same time pursuing the broader life setting in which symptoms occur.

Show interest in and commitment to the patient.
Introduce self, address patient by name, attend to physical comfort, elicit the patient's view of the problem, have good eye contact.

Facilitate communication.
Allow patient to give his own story of illness, use a balance of open-ended and closed-ended techniques, use nonbiasing questions, seek clarification of vague or ambiguous data, use empathy where appropriate, nonjudgmental, respect the patient, arrange space comfortably, posture communicates interest, quiet attention.

Avoid hindering behavior.
Avoid technical language, injecting biases, false or premature reassurance, frequent interrupting, posture communicates disinterest, not listening, reading chart or writing note during interview, allowing interruption, closed posture.

Table 4.2   Examples of skills necessary for good interviewing technique (cont.)

Assess barriers to communication (deafness, child, *etc.*).

Check barriers and compensate: talk louder, get interpreter.

Observe verbal and nonverbal signs of barriers at outset.

Inquire in an open-ended way about affect.

Negotiation and contracting share responsibility for patient care.

Check patient's understanding of diagnosis and treatment plan.

CHAPTER 5

*Communicating Through the
Medical Record*

Communicating through the medical record is a crucial aspect of medical care. According to a recent survey of U.S. medical schools, write-up of the patient history and physical examination, progress note, and the discharge summary were among the five most important types of writing for physicians to learn (Yanoff 1988). Yet only 43 of the 100 responding schools offered a course or program that specifically taught physicians how to write up a history and a physical examination; even fewer taught how to write progress notes; and, only eight gave instruction on writing discharge summaries.

During ward rotations students and residents have the greatest opportunity to learn about the critical role of the chart in the delivery of health care. Unfortunately, record-keeping is generally tedious, unexciting, and often viewed as the least important aspect of a patient's care, particularly during emergencies or unexpected events. Yet, without written information regarding the course of a patient's illness, future decisions cannot be appropriately made, and evaluation of past care is impossible. It is imperative for physicians to pay meticulous attention to their record-keeping. Although it is not an exciting part of the ward attending's jobs to teach students about medical records, it is during the ward experience that this skill is best learned. Table 5.1 outlines the role of the attending in this task.

The uses of the medical record are diverse, including provision of information about patients and their care, and communication among care providers. In more recent years it has become a tool for evaluation in quality assurance and risk management. It is increasingly used as a legal document. The varied uses of the medical record are listed in Table 5.2 (adapted from Huffman 1972).

Studies of the validity of content in the medical record compared to the interaction between patients and physician indicate that a large percentage of the information elicited is not documented in charts (Romm 1981; Moran 1988; Woolliscroft 1984). Recording is relatively complete for the chief complaint and the history of the patient's present illness, but poor for social, family, and other past medical history. The need for documentation also varies with the level of the medical learners and the purpose for which their write-ups is used. The medical student write-up must show to the attending physician what he has learned, as well as indicating that he is capable of including the pertinent information. As they mature, medical learners must produce more concise write-ups that conform more to the expected format. Admission notes written by the supervisory resident must indicate not only that he understands the patient and the medical issues, but also that he has provided adequate guidance for the student or resident. This note should also indicate the expected course of the patient's disease, anticipated problems, and how they will be managed.

All students and residents must learn about necessary components of the medical record, how to write them, and what the common pitfalls are. According to Sanders (1987) there are four essential characteristics of a good hospital medical chart: completeness, objectivity, consistency, and accuracy. Charts should include the following:

Admitting history: The date and time should be recorded. The admitting history includes the patient's name, and the name of the informant and an assessment of the informant's reliability. Preferably, names of persons to contact and telephone numbers should be listed in case of an acute change in the patient's condition or need for permission for procedures if the patient is not competent to do so. The history should identify the patient's chief complaint, and other complaints, including the duration of symptoms and a clear, chronologic, description of the illness. Other information to be included are family history, review of systems, past medical history, allergies and adverse reactions to medications, and the names and dosages of current medications.

A social history including living situation, history of drug or alcohol use, psychiatric conditions, and occupation are also critical, but often omitted because they are thought to be sensitive issues. Either during the hospitalization, or upon discussion of the patient with the attending, it may become obvious that portions of the admission history are inaccurate. Significant revisions of the history should be noted in the chart.

The record of a complete physical examination must include pertinent negative findings and should note differences between the patient's complaints and physical findings, *e.g.* the patient complains of abdominal pain, but the examination reveals no guarding or other indication of tenderness. The surname of the writer should be printed beside the signature.

Physician's orders: Clear, concise orders facilitate communications with other hospital staff. Orders should be specific, including what types of problems require notification of the physician; *e.g.* notification if temperature or blood pressure is greater than a specific value. One of the most common problems in charting is legibility of handwriting (White 1986). It is particularly critical that orders be absolutely legible, that drug dosages be checked, *particularly for decimal points*, and that the information be accurately transferred from the order sheet to the various entities, such as the pharmacy.

Progress notes: Progress notes should be concise and objective. The date and time of the note should be recorded, and again, the note should be signed with the surname printed alongside. Notes should be written in a timely manner that is in keeping with the condition of the patient and the management plan. If, for example, "frequent observation" is listed as part of the patient's management, brief notes should be written to indicate that this was done and the result of the observation.

Notes should be written any time there is a significant change in the patient's condition, and if the physician is called by the nurse, the patient, or the family to see the patient. Use of the SOAP format is recommended: S=subjective data, statements by the patient regarding how he feels; O=objective findings, including the physical examination and the results of laboratory tests or procedures; A=assessment of the patient's medical condition and problems; and P=plans for further diagnosis or treatment. Although the foregoing explanation of SOAP may seem very elementary, it illustrates avoidance of one of the common errors in charting: abbreviations.

Only widely recognized abbreviations should be used (NaPier 1989). Abbreviations that may commonly be used in one specialty may be either completely unknown to others, or may mean something completely different.

All procedures performed should be documented. A note should be written with the date and time of the procedure, a description of the procedure, the patient's response, and any complications.

Documentation of any procedures recommended but refused by the patient: If a procedure is recommended, but refused, a note must be written describing why the procedure was recommended, and why the patient refused it.

Operative Reports and discharge summaries: The importance of accurate and complete discharge summaries and operative reports is often underestimated (Mageean 1986). One of the most important aspects of operative reports and discharge summaries is that they be completed in a timely fashion. Not only can a report dictated long after a procedure or a hospitalization be discounted as not reflective of the situation at the time, a delay in the dictation hinders communication of vital information to the patient's primary care physician. It now also affects hospital reimbursement.

Residents and students should be taught to manage their time so that reports and summaries are dictated the day of the procedure or discharge. Information in the discharge summary includes: *identifying data* to include the patient's full name, address, date of birth, hospital number, and the name and address of the primary care physician who will provide on-going care; *clinical data* to include date of admission and discharge, and the date of the report; *admission data,* including the presenting symptoms, a synopsis of the admission history and the past medical history, medications on admission, and abnormalities on the physical examination. A summary of test results, procedures, and consultations should also be listed. *Management data* should include a brief description of the hospital course, what treatments were instigated and the patient's response, the prognosis of the illness, the expected course, and arrangements for follow-up.

Information regarding plans for follow-up is perhaps the most critical part of the discharge summary and needs to be both specific and concise. If further testing is needed, this should be outlined, with a discussion of who should do the testing, and when it should be done. If the patient is to see other consultants or needs to return to the hospital, the names of the consultants and the time when the patient is expected to return should be included. All medications that the patient is taking at discharge should be listed. When the dictated discharge summary has been typed, it should be *carefully proofread!* A copy of the discharge summary should be promptly sent to the patient's primary care physician and any consultants who will be seeing the patient after discharge.

Learning how to read the medical record and respond to the information contained in the record is an important part of the process of documentation of patient care. Students and residents need to learn to read the nurses' notes. Should there be discrepancies between the nurses' notes and their own observations, these should be noted in the chart. If there are comments in those notes that require action, *e.g.* the nurse writes that the patient was having difficulty breathing, this fact and the resident's assessment and plan for addressing the problem should be indicated in the chart.

Students and residents must also learn to read all written laboratory, radiology, and pathology reports. Often physicians will look at x-rays with the radiologist and receive a verbal report. Unfortunately, it is not uncommon for the final, written, report to have different information than what was given verbally. These discrepancies can sometimes be large, and often critical to the patient's care. The same is true for consultations. In the hospital setting, it is not uncommon for the students and residents to either be present at the time of consultation or to speak personally with the consultant. Again, the final written report may differ significantly from the verbal discussion.

If treatment is instituted or changed after a verbal discussion with a consultant, but before the report has been written, the discussion should be noted. If the attending physician does not agree with the recommendations of the consultant, this must be written with a statement regarding why a conclusion was reached, and that this information was presented to the patient. The patient's response and decision regarding choice of treatment should be documented.

Table 5.3 lists the most common mistakes that are made in charting and hazards that should be avoided (Sanders 1987; NaPier 1989). Among the most common and most important is illegibility. White and Beary (1986) screened 50 attending physician and resident progress notes for number of illegible words, reading time, comprehensibility of content, and legibility of signature. Fully 89 percent of the signatures were illegible, thus the need for printing the surname beside the signature, as recommended above, is essential. A mean of 16 percent of the words were illegible. Poor handwriting made increased reading time necessary in 42 percent of all charts, and decreased comprehension in 42 percent. The magnitude of the problem is obviously great. It is not the attending's responsibility to teach handwriting to students and residents, but he at least needs to serve as a good role-model. He should return illegible notes and work-ups, insisting that they be written in a way that they can be read.

Often there have been mistakes made in writing the medical record. The record should never be deliberately altered. Errors should be crossed out with a single line through the incorrect entry. The original entry should still be visible and legible. The change should be dated, timed, and initialed.

Objective language should be used and criticism of others avoided. Lawsuits have been instituted because of information that was inappropriately included in a chart. If there has been a lapse in care, communication with the person responsible should be direct. This is not to say that mistakes made during the hospitalization should be hidden. In fact, it is extremely important that they be documented. Sensitive issues, such as the fact that the patient was inebriated should not be avoided, but should be written in an objective fashion. NaPier suggests the following in this situation: "The patient smelled of alcohol, stumbled as he walked, and admitted consuming a fifth of Tequila this afternoon."

Teaching students and residents about medical records and their importance is not easy, and certainly not as much fun as teaching about diseases and their management. This information, however, is essential in their education and the ward experience is the best place to learn it. To assist attendings in this endeavor, a list of the responsibilities of attending's for the medical record and a check list to use when reviewing student and resident charts are included in tables 5.4 and 5.5 (adapted from Morrison S: The Ideal Chart).

Table 5.1 Attending's role in teaching communication through charting

1. Insist on legibility. Be a good role-model. Return illegible charts to students and residents to be re-written.

2. Teach appropriate charting either through lecture or by frequent review of resident and student charts.

3. Review write-ups of students for content, knowledge, accuracy, and objectivity.

4. Insist on timeliness for dictation of operative or procedural r.

Table 5.2 Purpose of the medical record

Documentation of the patient's illness and medical treatment.

Communication between the physician and other professionals.

Provision of continuity of care by hospital or medical staff personnel.

Provision of data for third parties, other physicians and hospitals, insurance companies or prepayment agencies, compensation carriers, attorneys, government agencies, and quality of assurance/risk management committees.

Provision of data to assist in protecting the legal interest of the patient, the hospital, and medical staff.

Provision of clinical data for research, study, and education.

adapted from: Huffman EK: *Medical Record Management.* Berwn, Illinois: Physicians' Record Company, 1972: p.123.

Table 5.3 Hazards to avoid: common errors in documentation in the medical chart

1. Illegible writing
2. Alterations
3. Use of abbreviations
4. Criticism of others
5. Subjective remarks
6. Omission of sensitive information
7. Lack of appropriate or timely documentation of procedures
8. Documentation of procedures recommended, but refused by the patient
9. Lack of proofreading of dictated medical records

Table 5.4   Responsibilities of the attending physician for the medical record

1. Diagnosis on the admission and discharge summaries are recorded and are accurate. Symbols and abbreviation should be avoided.

2. All entries are dated and signed and the entries of house officers countersigned as required by the Joint Commission on Accreditation of Hospitals.

3. The report of the history and physical examination is complete and contains all pertinent positive and negative findings.

4. Progress notes give a chronological picture and analysis of the clinical course of the patient. The frequency with which they are made is determined by the condition of the patient.

5. The results of all diagnostic laboratory and x-ray procedures are recorded, dated, and properly signed.

6. Consultations have been held in accordance with medical staff bylaws and have been adequately recorded and signed. Consultation should include consultant's findings on physical examination of the patient as well as his opinion and recommendations. If the attending has not followed the consultant's recommendations this is noted and explained.

7. Nurses' notes and entries by allied health personnel contain pertinent observations as well as a record of any treatment.

8. That a discharge summary is written or dictated at the time of discharge.

Table 5.5   Checklist for attendings when reviewing students' and residents' charts

1. Is there a completed history and physical promptly written upon admission, particularly in emergency cases?

2. Is there a clear description of the clinical problem in the admission note?

3. Is there a plan for work-up and management?

4. Are there progress notes at intervals to explain the patient's course, dated and timed, and written with a frequency that is in keeping with the progress of the patient's disease?

5. Do the progress notes document clearly the patient's status, including changes or complications?

6. Are reasons for specific treatments documented?

7. Are there continued comments and documentation on patient's response to therapy?

8. Are there justifications for special tests ordered and are review of test results included?

9. Is an analytic, clear view of the hospital course, response to treatment, and outcome documented? Does this documentation justify each day that the patient stays in the hospital?

10. Is there a final listing of diagnoses and/or procedures that is accurate and complete?

11. Is there documentation of discharge planning and follow-up including medications, tests to be completed or followed-up on an outpatient basis, and when and to whom the patient is to go for follow-up?

CHAPTER 6

Teaching Medical Procedures

When Dr. George L. Engel, a professor of psychiatry and medicine at the University of Rochester, visits other medical schools, he routinely asks students and residents whether, since their introduction to interviewing in their freshmen or sophomore years, their patient interviews have ever been critiqued. "More often than not, I get a stare of misbelief, students and residents appearing incredulous that such a teaching arrangement could even exist" (1982, p. 12). In response to the apparent lack of direct supervision of basic medical skills, such as learning how to interview a patient, Engel has compared medicine to music:

> Learning how to interview a patient is as basic to medicine as learning how to play an instrument is to music.... If musicians learned to play their instruments as physicians learn to interview patients, the procedure would consist of presenting in a lecture or maybe a demonstration or two

the theory and mechanisms of music-producing ability of the instrument, then handing the student an unfamiliar instrument and telling him to produce a melody. The instructor, of course, would not be present to observe or listen to the student's efforts but would be satisfied with the student's subsequent report of what came out of the instrument (p. 12).

The question raised by Engel is, do we teach basic skills, like interviewing, without direct observation? Our own experience suggests the answer is, "Not always, but often." This view was shared by Collins and colleagues at the Montreal Children's Hospital who observed and videotaped pediatric ward rounds. They reported that, "There was little attempt...to challenge, stimulate, encourage or correct the trainees or to demonstrate or watch them demonstrate proper skills and techniques" (1978, p. 430). Thus, we feel that ward attendings can provide an important service by scheduling two opportunities to observe each medical student interviewing and examining a patient. This can be done once in the first week and once in the last week of the rotation. In addition, they should identify medical procedures relevant to their hospital service and schedule time to teach these.

We begin with the premise that ward attendings may take medical procedures for granted. The problem is that when people become experts, they may forget what it is like to be a novice. A.T. Welford, a pioneer in the field of skilled human performance, pointed out that thoroughly performed actions tend to become automatic in the sense that they are done without conscious control (1976). When this occurs to instructors, they may find it difficult to teach procedures. This problem was identified by W. Lewis Robinson, vice president of industrial training for Industrial Correspondence Schools, who commented that a problem with many industrial training programs is that instructors are often too competent to do a good job. They may be so advanced in their own work that they have become oblivious to the needs of the novice. In a sense, they are too competent to be instructors:

> They know their jobs so well that they no longer have to think about what they are doing. They have arrived at the point where they can perform a given task unconsciously. They are competent, but they are unconsciously competent, and that's what makes them poor instructors. They no longer are conscious of the step-by-step process behind the successful completion of the task. Therefore, they cannot communicate properly to a trainee–to an individual who is consciously incompetent–about what it takes to do the job (*Personnel Journal* 1974).

The need for the teacher to join the learner at his stage of competence is highlighted in the teaching of the game of chess. Imagine an eight-year old teaching another eight-year old how to play chess. In about ten minutes they can be having an enjoyable game. The teacher knows the right language to use and the learner never has the slightest doubt that he can soon grasp the game. But, watch an adult chess expert try to teach another adult. The expert knows far too much and discusses all the scientific names for the openings, middle game, and the closing. The beginner becomes far too confused, unsure, and intimidated to learn such a complicated game.

This problem occurs on ward rounds when procedures are taught according to the "See one. Do one. Teach one." dictum. Instead, as described by Dr. Perri Klass (1987) when she was shown how to draw arterial blood, what may occur is "See three. Try four. Miss them all." She commented is her book, *Four Years as Medical Student: A Not Entirely Benign Procedure*, "For the medical student, life is full of opportunities to show off your ignorance." Under more favorable conditions, Dr. Melvin Konner (1987) learned how to perform intubation from anesthesiologist, Dr. Nina Hamedeh: "She was always friendly to me, always helpful, and–whatever I did–full of praise. She simply knew how to manage my ignorance into competence. By the end of the first day I had done three intubations, each as successful as the first." Unfortunately, after bungling two lumbar punctures on his neurology rotation, Dr. Konner became familiar with what housestaff called The Galen Rule of Teaching: "See one. Screw one. Do one."

The need to be friendly and to view the skill from the learner's viewpoint is understood in the world of dog sled racing. Yvan Binette, a Quebec dog sled driver commented that, "To get a dog to run for you, you have to be real friendly. You have to think like a dog. You have to lie down on all fours to see what the world looks like to a dog..." We think that to teach medical procedures, it also helps to be real friendly and to look at the world through the eyes of the medical student or resident.

Teaching a procedure is itself a procedure. To help you become "consciously competent" at this teaching skill, we have adapted the work of Marsha Prater, an educational specialist at the Memorial Medical Center in Springfield, Massachusetts, who has broken down the teaching of a psychomotor skill into its component steps (1991). According to Prater, medical procedures have three characteristics which distinguish them somewhat from verbal skills. First, they represent a chain of motor responses (muscle movements). Secondly, they involve the coordination of hand and eye movements (rather than tongue and eye movements as in verbal skills). Thirdly, they require the organization of response chains (sub-tasks or subroutines) into complex response patterns. It is easy to see how the insertion of a bladder catheter incorporates these three characteristics. It certainly involves both gross and fine body movements in manipulating equipment and setting up a sterile field; it

requires coordination of hand movements and visual perceptions to locate the urinary meatus and insert a catheter into the urethra; and it incorporates various sub-tasks
(such as putting on sterile gloves and appropriately prep-
ping the perineum) into the successful completion of the
procedure.

During an initial "cognitive" phase, individuals
intellectualize and analyze the skill to be performed. In
the "fixation" phase, the response patterns of performing
the skill are practiced until the correct response behaviors
are "fixed" and the chances of making errors are significantly reduced. And finally, the individual enters the
"autonomous" phase (becomes an "expert") which is characterized by increasing speed of performance and resis-
tance to external distractions. These phases are well-
illustrated by the novice student who needs to "talk himself through" the steps of tying surgical knots and the
practiced surgeon whose hands move smoothly with little or no conscious attention to the individual movements
which make up the complex task.

Also, according to Prater, research has identified
three important conditions which influence skill learning:
contiguity, practice and feedback. Contiguity is the
occurrence of the proper sequence and appropriate timing of motor responses without which the skill cannot be
performed. For example, in performing the skill of
suture removal, the student must first cut the suture
before attempting to pull it through the skin. Attempting

to pull on the suture and remove it without cutting the knot first prevents the successful completion of the skill.

The second important condition for learning psychomotor skills is practice. Practice allows for the rehearsing and fixation of the motor responses necessary for completion of the skill. The more closely the conditions of practice approach the conditions under which the skill will be used, the more effective is the practice. How much practice is necessary to adequately "learn" a skill is dependent upon the ability of the student and the complexity of the skill. Thus, due to the difficulty of the skill, it will usually take more practice to learn to insert an arterial catheter than it does to learn to start a peripheral intravenous catheter.

Feedback is the third condition influencing psychomotor skill learning. It is also the single most important variable governing the acquisition of skills. Feedback involves more than merely telling a student whether he performed the procedure correctly or not. It is more accurately defined as the process of providing learners information about current performance in order that they may improve their performance in the future. Without feedback, mistakes go uncorrected, good performance is not reinforced and clinical competence is achieved empirically or not at all.

As Prater suggests, it is unrealistic to expect students to learn medical procedures skills simply by reading or hearing about them. And yet, all too often the techniques used for imparting cognitive data to students are also used for teaching psychomotor skills. Lectures, videotapes, blackboard demonstrations and procedure manuals may be used to give students the background knowledge of indications, contraindications, potential complications and necessary equipment used for procedures, but learning to perform procedures requires "hands on" practice and feedback.

Thus, learning medical procedures requires a "patient" on which to practice and an "instructor" to provide feedback to students on their performance. "Patients" may take various forms such as human volunteers (*i.e.* fellow medical students) and simulated patients as well as actual patients. Likewise, various "instructors" can be utilized, from allied health personnel to nurses and residents. The one item that cannot be substituted, however, is the opportunity for students to practice and perfect their skill performance. This is perhaps best (but not always most easily) accomplished by providing a concentrated time devoted to learning technical skills at a patient's bedside under the supervision of an experienced clinician.

When teaching students or residents medical procedures skills, several steps should be followed. The teaching can be divided into three basic phases: introductory, practice, perfecting. The introductory steps are used to help the student and residents intellectualize the skill and develop a mental plan for performance. The practice steps facilitate learning the skill by providing students and residents with immediate feedback on their behavior, thus eliminating errors and strengthening correct responses. Finally, the perfecting phase may continue for an extended period of time (*i.e.* over the entire clerkship) as students and residents perform the skill under realistic conditions and gain in speed and precision.

Due to the advancement of medical technology in recent years, the need for medical students and residents to become proficient in medical procedures is increasing. Traditionally, however, students have learned skills in a haphazard and unstructured manner. This approach can leave them ill-prepared to handle many clinical situations as interns and residents. An understanding of how individuals learn psychomotor skills is important in developing a more effective approach to teach such skills. Students need to develop a mental plan for performance of the skill, be given numerous practice opportunities under realistic performance conditions, be provided immediate informational feedback to eliminate errors and reinforce correct responses, and develop an ability to independently evaluate their performance to encourage continued improvement.

Earlier in this chapter, we reported the finding of Collins *et al.* that attending physicians did not routinely watch medical students perform medical skills and techniques. In the same study, questionnaire results showed that, while both medical students and ward attendings agreed that there were a number of skills which should be assessed on rounds, they did not agree as to whether this was occurring. On the questionnaire, 79 percent of the attending physicians felt that they used ward rounds to assess such performance, whereas only 46 percent of the students perceived this to be happening (1978). If an attending physician evaluates students, but they do not know they were being evaluated, then was there, in fact, an evaluation? This is like the, "If a tree falls in the forest..." paradox. Because of its importance to medical education, assessment and feedback will be addressed in chapter eight and evaluation in chapter nine. But, first, it will be helpful to address how to manage mistakes which might require immediate intervention.

CHAPTER 7

Managing Medical Mistakes

Ultimately...every physician must reconcile his responsibility for peoples' lives with the inevitability of making mistakes.... The age of the physician does not guarantee that mistakes will be avoided. Mistakes are distressing to the oldest as well as the youngest physician, both of whom must realize that even the most experienced and wisest of clinicians are subject to error. Indeed, clinical wisdom involves in part the acceptance of this fact (Dubovsky and Schrier 1983).

Of the attitudes, beliefs, and values that a ward attending can effect, one of the most important is teaching medical learners what to do when a mistake has been made. Mistakes are inevitable; they come in all sizes: large, small, inconsequential, and devastating. Wu *et al.* in asking whether house officers learn from their mistakes, began their article with a quotation from Goethe that succinctly describes the role of teaching and learning from errors (1991):

> The most fruitful lesson is the conquest of
> one's own error. Whoever refuses to admit
> error may be a great scholar, but he is not a
> great learner. Whoever is ashamed of error
> will struggle against recognizing and
> admitting it, which means that he struggles
> against his greatest inward gain.

Mistakes can be powerful, formative experiences, and, ideally, could be used as teaching tools by medical educators. However, this is an extremely difficult task, for medical errors always have the potential to be devastating to both the one who makes the mistake and the unfortunate patient who has received inappropriate care. In their study, Wu *et al.* found that only 54 percent of the time did residents discuss significant mistakes with their attending physicians, and only 24 percent shared this information with either the patient or his family. This was the case despite the fact that 90 percent of the mistakes resulted in serious adverse patient outcomes, including death in 31 percent. Importantly, residents who accepted their mistakes and were able to discuss them were more likely to report constructive changes in their practices when compared with residents who felt the institution to be judgmental.

Because of the type of work, the complexity of the patients, and the setting, mistakes are probably both more likely to be made and more likely to be detected during rotations on wards or in intensive care units. Thus, during an attending rotation, it is very likely that the situation will arise in which a potentially serious error has been made. Such situations create anxiety, not only for the medical learner who has made the error, but also for the attending, who may be legally responsible for the consequences of the error, and is also responsible for the education and acculturation of the learner who has, in this case, failed.

To manage such situations well, the attending must be a consummate teacher, using the principles that have already been discussed in the chapters of this book. The following is an outline of one method for systematically dealing with mistakes. This can help create patterns of behaviors among medical learners that will allow them to use their mistakes as learning experiences.

Step One: Create an atmosphere that is non-threatening and nonjudgmental, so that open discussion of mistakes can occur.

> At some point we must bring our mistakes out of the closet. We need to give ourselves permission to recognize our errors and their consequences. We need to find healthy ways to deal with our emotional responses to those errors. Our profession is difficult enough without our having to wear the yoke of perfection (Hifiker 1984).

One of the first ways to create an open communications system is by anticipating problems. Certainly, an attending can make the assumption that at some point during his teaching rotation errors will occur. Discuss this with the learners at the very beginning of the rotation, outlining what the student should do if he feels that he has made an error. An explanation that early discovery and discussion of errors may make remedial intervention possible should motivate the learners to communicate their concerns with the attending. The discussion should be done in a nonjudgmental tone, not tolerating carelessness or errors, but accepting the fact that mistakes are common, that those who make them do so unintentionally and are not "bad people," and that the most important aspects of mistakes are recognizing them and addressing the consequences.

One of the methods for creating a relatively non-threatening environment is for the attending to use the previously discussed "professional intimacy" skills to talk about the mistake: what did the student or resident do and how does he feel about it? This can then set the stage for open communications, that may, in fact, decrease the chances that errors will occur.

Step two: Ensure that supervision is adequate so that errors are detected.

In order to use mistakes as learning experiences, errors must be detected. Often in medicine, there are very differing opinions about medical management. These differences are not errors, but should a poor outcome be the result of a controversial decision, this can be openly discussed in the same manner as mistakes. The attending must supervise the work of the senior resident, ensuring that the quality of the resident's work is adequate, that his judgement is sound, and that he can detect errors. It is then the responsibility of the resident to oversee the day-to-day work of the junior residents and students. The next step is to ensure that a communication system is in place, so that the attending is informed of potential errors. He must determine if there actually was a mistake, why the mistake was made, and what needs to be done.

If the attending is fortunate, the first detected mistake will either be a minor one, or one which is not associated with an adverse medical outcome. This gives the attending and the supervisory resident the opportunity to "practice" the system for dealing with mistakes under circumstances that are not terribly threatening. Any system will work more effectively at times when there is little or no emotional stress.

Step three: Determine the cause of the error.

Just as with "accidents," mistakes are not random. The actual cause of medical errors can generally be classified into one of three categories: inexperience, job overload, and case complexity. There is a fourth category of mistakes, however, that requires a great deal more remediation. Sometimes mistakes are made because a medical learner's attitudes are not compatible with the practice of medicine. In chapter three, ten attitudes that are core to a medical learner's ability to solve medical problems were listed: being careful, attentive, curious, skeptical, honest, objective, receptive to new ideas, systematic, decisive and persistent. If the student's or resident's attitude is problematic, it is unlikely that he will learn from his error, and his mistakes may well become repetitive. If after a discussion of the issue, the attending is convinced that the learner's attitude is inappropriate (e.g. he is dishonest and will not take responsibility for the mistake), more drastic steps, such as informing the appropriate medical school authority or the residency director, must be taken.

Fortunately, these issues are rare. Most learners will be frightened by their errors, remorseful, and highly motivated to learn what they can do to avoid future errors. The attending can sit down with the learner and objectively review the facts to determine the cause of the error. Every attempt should be made to separate the action (mistake) from the person, so that the discussion will be as non-threatening as possible.

Using one of the basic principles of giving feedback, the attending should start with the learner by asking him what he thought, why he thought the error occurred, and what the current course of action should be. This can give the attending insight into the learner's ability for "self-correction."

By the end of the discussion, there should be agreement regarding the mistake: why it happened, what the consequences of the error were, and what remediation needs to be done, both for the patient and for the resident. Then, cooperatively, the learner and the attending must decide how widely to share this experience. Is this mistake so personal and unique that the learning experience will only be meaningful to the resident who made the error, or is this a more common mistake that potentially every physician might make? If it is a mistake that should be shared, how this will be done and how the learner still protected emotionally should be planned. This process can produce "professional intimacy" and may help the learner not only deal with his own mistakes better in the future, but also demonstrate ways he can help others in turn.

All hospitals now have quality assurance, risk management committees. Generally, residents are not involved with the review of errors that these committees do, because the attending is the legally responsible party. However, all physicians must learn how to relate to such committees. The attending should discuss with the resident what will happen administratively from this point on, and should share with him the eventual reports from the committee.

Step four: Determine a course of action for remediation.

There are two aspects to remediation: that for the patient and that for the resident. Decisions must be made regarding changes in the medical management of the patients, what to inform the patient and the family about the error that has been made, and notification of hospital administrators who are responsible for risk management. All of these steps may not need to be taken if a mistake is trivial, or results in no complication to the patients. However, as pointed out above, inconsequential mistakes can be used to demonstrate what needs to be done should a serious error occur. This can offer the opportunity for residents to learn how to discuss errors with patients and families. They will probably be surprised to learn that most patients, particularly if no harm has been done, will be quite open and sympathetic to the physician who is honestly describing his limitations.

Remediation for the resident depends upon the cause of the error. Situational errors, such as fatigue, must be addressed. Sometimes, the problem is programmatic. However, it may be that a given resident does not work efficiently or well when stressed to a lesser degree than others. If he is unable to function in situations that are essential to his chosen field, he may need career counseling. For most residents, they simply need to learn to recognize their limits, learn to ask for help, and how to get it. Remediation for mistakes of inexperience and also those that are the result of complexity of the case may also be programmatic or individual.

If the system of supervision is inadequate, the program needs to be adjusted to ensure that residents can get assistance. Individual problems include not recognizing limitations, failure to communicate, confusion regarding whom to call, and lack of knowledge. Steps that can be taken include closer supervision of the learner's work, with constant discussions regarding decision-making, review of communication principles and systems, and assigned reading. Case complexity can be addressed by assigning the resident similar cases that have fewer problems, so that he can learn in a step-wise and less anxiety-producing manner (matching responsibility and independence with knowledge and ability, as discussed in Stritter's "Learning Vector," chapter one).

Step five: Address the emotional needs of the learner.

Even the language used at medical centers creates an atmosphere that makes the emotional impact of errors potentially devastating. How often is prior management of patients highly criticized? The terms for the primary care physicians who refer their patients are derogatory: "LMD" (Local Medical Doctor) and "PMD" (Private Medical Doctor) are commonly heard being spoken in a tone of voice that allows no question regarding the quality of the care or the person responsible for it. Unfortunately, students and residents at the medical center do not see the cases that the local physician has managed successfully. They also have not been exposed to the circumstances of practice away from the medical center. The harsh judgements that are made often come from the unconscious realization that every physician is separated from mistakes only by extreme care and a bit of good luck.

This will not create an environment that is conducive to emotional support for residents when they have made a mistake. The first step in assisting residents with their emotions, is to teach them to be more understanding and sympathetic to others. They must learn to separate the person from the deed. This can only be done by abolishing such derogatory terms as "PMD" from our medical language. They can be taught to analyze the prehospital management of referred patients in an objective, rather than a judgmental manner. If a mistake was made in patient management, it can be discussed so that the cause of the error is determined, and a hypothetical remediation plan developed. Finally, the attending can ask the learners, "How do you think you would have felt if this had been your patient and you had made this error?"

If an environment that is non-threatening has already been established, the emotional aspects of dealing with a mistake will be easier for a resident than it might be. However, the attending should privately discuss with the resident how he feels, how much distress and guilt he has, and what type of personal support system he has. Occasionally, a resident will be so distressed that outside help and counselling will be needed. Usually, an open, understanding discussion with the attending with an invitation to return for further discussion if necessary will suffice.

Certainly, management of mistakes is among the most challenging of all teaching situations. If the attending is able to function well in this capacity, he has probably mastered all the techniques discussed in this book. Even though the situations are anxiety producing for all involved, they can be highly rewarding if appropriately managed. Mistakes have a way of making that forty-day month seem like sixty, but, if the attending has helped even one physician learn to "self-correct," learn from his errors, and not repeat them, the extra days are worth it!

The Marquis of Halifax claimed that if we knew "what men are most apt to remember, we might know what they are most apt to do." It makes sense to us that if an attending physician were aware of a medical student's or resident's fund of knowledge, he would be able to anticipate medical mistakes, at least some of the time. Since, for a specific medical problem, a learner may or may not be knowledgeable and the teacher may or may not be aware which is the case, Whitman and Schwenk (1984) addressed four scenarios in their handbook for clinical preceptors:

1. The learner knows, and the teacher knows he knows! This is shared knowledge. For example, you may be aware that the medical student knows the signs and symptoms of bronchial asthma.

2. The learner knows, but the teacher does not know he knows! This is hidden knowledge...hidden from the teacher. For example, you may not be aware

that the medical student also knows the signs and symptoms of respiratory acidosis.

3. The learner does not know, but teacher knows he does not know! This is an area of known needs... known to the teacher. For example, you may be aware that the medical student does not appreciate the importance of teaching asthmatic children to recognize their trigger factors.

4. The learner does not know, and the teacher does not know that! This is an area of unknown needs... unknown to the teacher and, perhaps, unknown to the learner who does not know what it is he does not know. For example, you may not be aware that the student does not know how to draw arterial blood.

If the attending physician assessed this student's knowledge or skill, it would be possible for him to target instruction at known needs and, by reducing the area of unknown needs, lower the possibility of medical mistakes. This does not mean that all known needs have to be addressed in one month. It does mean that the attending physician can protect the student (and patient) from making mistakes. This is one interpretation of the teacher defending his students statement made in the Introduction to this book.

In this chapter, we recommended ways of dealing with medical mistakes. Although it is unlikely that mistakes can be completely eliminated, we believe that some mistakes can be prevented. The key to prevention is assessing medical students and residents at the start of the month so that you have some estimate of their abilities and limits and giving feedback during the month so that they become aware of their strengths and weaknesses.

CHAPTER 8

Assessment and Feedback

On ward rounds, learning is a process of internally organizing new knowledge, attitudes and skills. The basis for this organization is a "diagnosis of inadequacy." Is there is a discrepancy between where the medical student is and where he wants to be? Since effective education requires that the learner, as well as the teacher, recognize this need, the diagnosis of inadequacy should be a collaborative process involving both of them. As noted by Leland Bradford, the co-founder of the National Training Laboratory (NTL) in Group Development, *"It is ineffectual for someone else to make the diagnosis for the learner— a frequent fault in education."*

Thus, diagnosis should include the *student's* motivations, desires, anxieties, insecurities, perceptions, *etc.* In addition, diagnosis depends upon having adequate data. Do medical teachers take the time to find out what students know and do not know, what attitudes, beliefs, and values are shared and not shared, and what the student's skill level is? In the field of education, the term assessment is used to describe this diagnostic process. In its derivation, the word assess means "to sit beside" or "to assist the judge" (Anderson *et al.* 1977). Thus, assessment requires first-hand gathering of data and fashioning these into an interpretation.

Reliable diagnosis of students, like diagnosis of patients, requires a two-way exchange of information, emotion, and meaning (Dodge 1983). In developing teaching skills, clinicians may find it helpful to recognize that clinical care and clinical teaching use the same set of communication skills, *e.g.* eliciting the concerns of another person, asking questions, and listening. *Thus, the key to assessing student needs, or, in other words, diagnosing inadequacies, is to treat the student as a patient, applying all the communication skills used every day in patient care.*

HELPFUL INTERACTIONS

There are many ways in which caring for patients and teaching students and residents are similar because both clinical care and clinical teaching are "service professions," sharing the aim of helping others. The role of the teacher as a helper is emphasized in the adult education literature. In a handbook for adult educators, *Helping Others Learn*, McLagan (1978) specifically defined the teacher's role in terms of *helping* learners (1) become motivated to learn, (2) effectively handle course materials, (3) develop new knowledge, attitude, and skills, and (4) apply what they have learned. One implication of this view is that the teacher is no longer responsible for the accomplishment of these four tasks–for the most part, the student is.

Thus, teaching and learning is a collaborative venture which depends upon teachers and learners sharing responsibility for programmatic success. In a study of clinical teaching, Tiberius and colleagues at the Medical School of the University of Toronto found that medical students respond much more enthusiastically to teachers whom they regard as interested in them and clinical teachers respond much more enthusiastically to students whom they perceive as eager to learn: "Interest, concern, commitment, enthusiasm, and eagerness are what make the process worthwhile for all the participants" (1989, p. 679).

In promoting helpful interactions, Gibb (1964) recognized that help is not always helpful! First of all, the learner must want to be helped. We are sure that you have known some medical students or residents who, in the words of Alexander Pope, "will never learn anything because they understand everything too soon" (Auden and Kronenberger 1981). Secondly, the learner must perceive that what is being offered is helpful. The problem here is that some teachers offer one type of help regardless of the needs of the learner. In a model developed by a communications specialist, Stuart Atkins (1981), there are four styles in offering help:

1. "Here are the pros and cons."
2. "What would you be comfortable doing?"
3. "Here's what I would do if I were you."
4. "I'm here if you need me."

The third barrier to help concerns the motivation of the helper. Does he wish to showcase his superior skill, control others, induce indebtedness, or establish dependency? With regard to establishing dependency, Gibb warned against setting out to train, advise, persuade, or indoctrinate others. This concern is shared by Dr. Thomas C. King, a Professor of Surgery at the College of Physicians and Surgeons of Columbia University:

> Any act of the clinician-teacher which reduces the resident's opportunity to gather his own information, analyze it, and use it to solve problems, undermines [the basic purpose of graduate medical education]. Our compulsion to give information in anticipation of need, to show off our intellectual skills, and to give right-answer conclusions is inimical to good teaching... (1991).

In order to help clinical teachers become more helpful, seven conditions suggested by Gibb are offered here:

1. *Reciprocal trust–* "Help" is most helpful when given in an atmosphere in which people have reciprocal feelings of confidence, warmth, and acceptance. When one feels that his worth as a person is valued he is able to place himself in psychological readiness to receive aid.

2. *Cooperative learning–* People are helpful to each other when they are engaged in a cooperative quest for learning…. Needs for help and impulses to give help arise out of the demands of the common cooperative task.

3. *Mutual growth–* The most permanent and significant help occurs in a relationship in which both members are continually growing, becoming, and seeking fulfillment.

4. *Reciprocal openness–* One of the most essential conditions for effective human learning is the opportunity for feedback or knowledge of progress.

5. *Shared problem solving–* The productive helping relationship focuses upon the problem to be solved…. The aspect of the behavior about which help is given should be seen as a shared problem, not as a defect to be remedied or as something to be solved by the helper as consultant.

6. *Autonomy–* The ideal relationship for helping is an interdependent one in which each person sees the other as both helper and recipient….

7. *Experimentation*– Tentativeness and innovative experimentation are characteristic of the most productive helping relationship. There is a sense of play, excitement, and fun in the common exploratory quest for new solutions to continually changing problems.

STUDENT RESPONSIBILITY

In assessing needs and promoting helpful interactions, ward attendings should recognize that medical students and residents are responsible for teaching themselves. As articulated by Neame and Powis,

> It must be acknowledged that a university course in medicine cannot hope to present to its students everything they need to know in order to practice a lifetime's career in the profession. Even were the course years longer, increasing the content of factual knowledge would not equip the graduate for the practice of medicine. In part this is due to the fact that medical knowledge is constantly changing or being reevaluated; in addition, facts alone cannot be correlated with practical application, and the process of how to use the facts is an essential part of the study and practice of medicine. It is essential, therefore, that an under-graduate medical course, among other things, teach

the students to take responsibility for and be able to structure their own learning (1981, p. 886).

The need for medical students to take more responsibility for their own education and to become independent learners was recognized in the AAMC General Professional Education of the Physician (GPEP) Report, *Physicians for the Twenty-First Century* (1984), which recommended that medical faculty should adopt evaluation methods to identify those students who have the ability to learn independently and provide opportunities for their further development of this skill. For those students who lack this ability, the GPEP Report recommended that the faculty challenge them to develop this ability.

Some medical schools anticipated the need to encourage students to take more responsibility for their own learning and, prior to the GPEP Report, instituted reforms in the first two years of the curriculum. Other schools have made these changes since then, and, yet others, are in the process of considering changes. According to a survey of medical educators from 127 U.S. medical schools, 97 percent of the respondents support or strongly support increasing the integration between the basic sciences and the clinical phases of medical student education and 86 percent support or strongly support decreasing the number of large lectures and increasing the time for independent study and interaction with faculty (Cantor *et al.* 1991).

We recommend that ward attendings learn what reforms have been made at their medical schools so that they can judge how well prepared students are to take responsibility for their own learning. If reforms are being discussed, ward attendings should consider participating in the process so that the students they are asked to supervise have learned how to learn. Ward attendings may find it encouraging that many schools have successfully implemented changes in the first two years aimed at helping students become more independent.

For example, in response to this long-recognized need for students to take more responsibility for their own learning, the Department of Pathology at the University of Medicine and Dentistry of New Jersey Robert Wood Johnson School of Medicine in 1986 adopted a major change in its second-year course. In the redesigned course, an instructor is assigned each week to cover that week's topic, providing guidelines, objectives, reading assignments, audiovisual material, and material for self-evaluation. There are only two lectures per week– one at the beginning to provide an overview and one at the end to provide a summation. Groups of twenty students each meet in three-hour sessions with an instructor to discuss the topic of the week and discuss one article presented by a student. In addition, students are encouraged to review on a computer questions provided by the national Group for Research in Pathology and by the faculty (Raskova, Martin, and Shea 1988).

The authors reported significant improvement on course examinations, an NBME shelf examination, and the pathology section of the NBME, and they had the impression that student adjustment to independent learning seemed to come gradually: "as the course progressed, most students developed new learning habits and self-confidence" (p. 487).

Also in response to the need to foster more student responsibility, the Department of Microbiology and Immunology at the University of Arkansas College of Medicine in 1987 changed their small-group clinical conferences that had been used to help second-year medical students apply their knowledge of pathogenic microbiology to clinical situations. Traditionally, during each session, a faculty member asked questions about microbiological laboratory procedures, presented a patient's case history, and posed questions pertaining to sequencing of laboratory tests and interpretation of results (Daly and Tysinger 1989).

In hopes of promoting students' independent learning and leadership skills by having them take responsibility for the teaching and learning activities of the conferences, student moderators were asked to present the case and pose questions. Faculty advisors met with student moderators in advance of the sessions to provide support and to serve as consultants in the conferences. Overall, the student and faculty evaluations of the conferences were very favorable. Based on student and faculty assessments, the authors learned that (1) students can handle more responsibility if they are given support to assume this new role and (2) faculty must work closely with students to identify the type and amount of support required.

The pathology faculty in New Jersey and the microbiology faculty in Arkansas have demonstrated that students can benefit from more responsibility. We realize that faculty elsewhere also have taken action. We encourage them to reflect upon what they have done and to publish the results so that others can be aware of their activities.

THERAPEUTIC EFFECT

In working with clinical teachers, we often hear that they are frustrated that there is not enough time to teach. Our understanding of this problem is that they want to accomplish too much. In this regard, it may be helpful to think of every encounter with a student or resident as an opportunity to have a therapeutic effect in the sense that this other person can be better off as a result of the encounter. In the context of patient care, clinicians understand and feel comfortable with the concept of the therapeutic effect. As a result of an encounter, is a patient better off in some, albeit, small way? For example, the clinician may provide reassurance, answer a single question, or do nothing more than schedule a follow up appointment. If clinicians expected "cure" to be the outcome of every encounter, the practice of medicine would be too frustrating.

Yet, when clinicians become clinical teachers, they unrealistically expect the educational equivalent of "cure," *i.e.*, they want to "teach it all." Instead, they should accept the same limitations as those of clinical care. As a result of an encounter with a student or resident, the clinical teacher may do as little as provide reassurance, answer a single question, or do nothing more than schedule a follow up session. If doing just one of those things is meeting a need of the learner, then the clinical teacher in an educational sense had a therapeutic effect!

Thus, every encounter with students and residents— which may occur over the telephone, in the hospital cafeteria, in the clinic coffee room, at the patient's bedside, along the hospital corridor, at morning report, or in the noon conference— provides an opportunity to have a therapeutic effect. In recognizing the value of incremental accomplishments, clinical teachers may feel less frustrated by the limitations of what they do. In addition, experienced clinicians realize that for some patients "cure" is not possible and recognize that "caring" is not a consolation prize for those who cannot be cured, but is a primary need. Similarly, we would encourage clinical teachers to recognize that showing that they care about students as individuals may meet a primary need. As stated by Kathrynn Thompson, a Clinical Associate at The Ohio State University,

> (What is important may be) an attitude for and about the student. This is an important quality that increasingly is lost in our society

of rapid social and technological changes. It is especially important in this system where students frequently feel that they are "lost in crowd." I believe that teaching involves a lot more than imparting knowledge. I believe you need to look at the whole student and care about each one personally (Verrier and Leser 1990).

FEEDBACK

Thus far, we have suggested that ward attendings...

• *assess needs so that the inadequacies of medical students and residents are addressed;*

• *promote helpful interactions so that there is collaboration;*

• *encourage students and residents to take responsibility for their own learning so that they can teach themselves; and*

• *aim at having a therapeutic effect so that students and residents potentially benefit from every interaction.*

In order for these processes to be successful, there is a need for continuous feedback. What is feedback and how do you give it? We believe that the answers to these two questions are crucial to the success of ward attending. The term, feedback, was originally used by rocket engineers in the 1940s. A rocket sent into space contains a mechanism that sends a signal back to Earth, where a steering apparatus receives these signals and makes adjustments if the rocket is off course (Hanson 1975). Norbert Weiner, the founder of the field of cybernetics, recognized that using feedback to change human performance was a type of learning (1950), and the psychologist, Kurt Lewin, helped to popularize the term, feedback, to describe the process of letting other persons know your perceptions of their behavior (Hanson 1975).

Of course, supervisors have always told subordinates what they they thought of their performance, and, when the field of educational psychology was dominated by stimulus and response, feedback was viewed as a form of reward or punishment called *"motivation"* feedback. Motivational feedback has the generalized effect of increasing or decreasing the likelihood that the behavior it follows will be repeated. Certainly, positive feedback is rewarding and negative feedback is punishing, and, as such, influences behavior. However, attending physicians should keep in mind that, in most cases, positive feedback is a more powerful motivator than negative (Tosti 1978).

Today, with the rise of the field of cognitive psychology, feedback also is viewed as a form of information. This view of feedback, known as *"informational"* or *"formative"* feedback, aims to guide or improve performance by shaping the target behavior toward a criterion (Tosti 1978). Rather than focusing simply on stimulus and response, psychologists today are interested in the characteristics of the person receiving as well as giving the feedback. For example, recipients perceive feedback differently as a function of self-esteem and other personal characteristics (Cathcart and Samovar 1989).

While the *motivational* nature of feedback is still important, the significance of its *informational* aspects was highlighted by a survey in which third and fourth year medical students perceived the feedback process as occurring less often than did faculty (Gil, Heins, and Jones 1984). Whether students are blind to the amount of feedback they receive or whether faculty exaggerate the amount that they provide could be addressed in an observational study. In any case, the discrepancies underscore the complexity of the feedback process (Sheehan 1985).

In numerous workshops for medical teachers, faculty have volunteered that they give too little positive feedback to medical students and residents, and have admitted difficulty giving negative feedback (Whitman 1985). This problem was cited by Dr. Jack Ende, Director of House Staff Training in the Department of Internal Medicine at the Boston University Medical Center:

> Not only are clinical skills infrequently observed, but when they are, the information so obtained does not get back where it can be most helpful– back to the trainees themselves. How widespread a concern is this? One needs only to poll a few medical students or house officers, or think back to

one's own training, to appreciate how little attention is given to feedback during clinical training (1983).

In addition, students complain that, at the start of a rotation, they are not told what is expected. In other words, they are not told ahead of time what success will look like. Sadler (1983) has coined the term, *"feedforward,"* to refer to prior specification of criteria so that students know what to aim for. According to Sadler, and we wholeheartedly agree, it is irresponsible for a teacher to tell a student *post facto*, "What I was really looking for was ..."

To improve clinical performance of medical students and residents, we recommend that attending physicians give both feedforward and feedback, providing what could be called a "Total Information Learning System" (TILS). The major assumption of TILS is that human beings are purposeful organisms who, if they know where they are supposed to be going, and, along the way, know whether or not they are on course, will make the necessary adjustments.

Although this notion of humans as purposeful learners makes sense today, prior to World War II, the field of educational psychology was dominated by hard-headed behaviorists who beat soft-hearted colleagues with the materialist claim that mental states and processes such as "being purposeful" do not really exist. Psychologists interested in mental events were put off by the argument that one could not point to a mental state such as "being purposeful." This view changed during World War II when psychologists worked closely with engineers who built purposeful machines based on the "servo-mechanism" principle:

> This general servo principle was used in the military to develop systems to point a big gun at a target....You want a mechanism that's going to be sensitive to any deviation between the actual position of the barrel of the gun and its intended position....The machine must be able to estimate the difference; as long as there's a difference, the system will feed that information back to keep the gun moving in such a way as to reduce the difference (Miller 1983).

Engineers could speak of machines as "goal seeking!" In the servo-system, the future position of that gun controls the present motion in a very real, perfectly intelligible way. This dynamic relationship between future and present events should be intuitive to clinicians who recognize that a patient's prognosis as well as diagnosis influences current treatment. In a similar vein, we hope that clinical teachers also recognize that feedforward and feedback can influence a student's or resident's clinical performance. The implication of the servo-mechanism for our Total Information Learning System is that medical students and residents will be purposeful when they set a target and hit it.

Setting a target was discussed by the AAMC Panel on the General Professional Education of the Physician (1984) which recommended that medical faculty should specify the clinical knowledge, skills, and values expected of medical students. Most residency directors (and residency review committees) would extend this feedforward recommendation to residency programs, as well. Thus, faculty should develop, with medical student and resident input, goals and objectives for each clinical rotation. We suspect that these goals and objectives have been prepared for most programs. But, are these shared with the students and residents at the start of each rotation? Perhaps, not.

In addition to sharing these goals and objectives with their learners, attending physicians also should ask for *their* goals and objectives. By asking medical students and residents to set their own targets, motivation will increase. This also is a good opportunity to begin the process of self-assessment by asking the medical students and residents to pre-establish criteria for success.

In order to hit the target, feedback to medical students and residents is essential. In providing feedback, attending physicians should use both positive and negative feedback. When performance is good, positive feedback is motivating as well as informative. In terms of motivation, it lets a person know what he is doing that is appreciated. Positive feedback may make a person feel good, which is rewarding, but it also should be informative. Specifically, what is this person doing right? The aim should be performance, not just feelings.

If you only make the person feel good, this is a compliment. While we are in favor of compliments, we would like attending physicians to be more specific so that medical students and residents get formative feedback. For example, "I like having you on my rotation!" is a compliment. On the other hand, "I like having you on my rotation because I can read your charts!" is an example of positive feedback.

When performance is not good, or needs to change in some way, negative feedback lets a person know what he is doing that is not appreciated. Negative feedback may make a person feed bad, which is punishing. If it is too threatening, the person may not be open to the informational aspect of the feedback. Instead, this person may become defensive, which could get in the way of improvement. In fact, in identifying the most helpful teaching behaviors, third and fourth year medical students cited the importance of "not belittling when wrong" (Stritter *et al.* 1975).

If an attending physician feels let down by a medical student or resident, he may wish to criticize him rather than to provide feedback. As pointed out by Hanson (1975), "Giving feedback effectively may depend on an individual's values and basic philosophy about himself, about his relationships with others, and about other people in general" (p. 153).

Since our philosophical aim is improvement, negative feedback is aimed at performance, not the person.

When a person feels criticized, his energy may go into self-protection rather than self-improvement. In a handout adapted from *A Handbook for Faculty Development* by Berquist and Phillips (1975) and developed by the Office of Medical Education Research and Development at Michigan State University, we are reminded that, "Feedback can be destructive when it only serves our own needs and fails to consider the needs of the person receiving it. Too often we give feedback because it makes us feel better or to give us the psychological advantage." Some attendings may ask, "Well, how about constructive criticism?" We find this phrase rarely helpful to the receiver.

The staff at Michigan State University also emphasize the need for feedback to be (1) descriptive rather than evaluative, (2) specific rather than general, and (3) focused on behavior rather than personality. Expanding upon their examples, we support the notion that it is better to say, "There seemed to be some patient discomfort when you used the ophthalmoscope," rather than, "Didn't anyone show you how to use an ophthalmoscope!" Similarly, it would be better to say, "When the patient indicated that he could not afford the medication, I did not see you respond," rather than to tell a student or resident that he is generally unresponsive to patient needs. In addition, we think it is more effective to show a student how to hold a scalpel than to tell him he is clumsy.

In providing feedback, positive or negative, we would like attending physicians to be selective and to focus on what is clinically significant. This means that you do not have to always "Tell it like it is." Instead, "Tell it like it is when **it is** important." On the other hand, we strongly support Pfeiffer and Jones's admonition: "Don't tell it like it isn't." In other words, what is to be avoided is deceiving medical students and residents.

Some attending physicians "tell it like it isn't" by giving medical students and residents negative feedback when positive was deserved. This is done in the name of "Let's keep them on their toes." We have actually been told by some attending physicians that positive feedback, even if deserved, will cause complacency. We could not disagree more. Our understanding of human nature is that, with positive feedback, most people work even harder.

Other attending physicians "tell it like it isn't" by giving medical students and residents positive feedback when negative was deserved or, by saying nothing about poor performance. This practice, known as "collusion" is characterized by an unwillingness to take risks and underestimates the ability of others to deal with openness (Pfeiffer and Jones 1972). Some attending physicians, understandably, want to get along and to be liked. Unfortunately, undeserved positive feedback or unspoken negative feedback merely sends the problem elsewhere.

The willingness to trust the ability of a student and the system to deal with honesty was epitomized by the attending physician who failed a sophomore medical student in the physical diagnosis course because, in taking a patient's history, his questions were too detailed, he allowed the patient to ramble, and he omitted key questions. In addition, the physical examination was awkward, unsystematic, and full of omissions. The student was given specific feedback and a week of intensive practice before re-testing. Later, when the student was in his first clinical rotation, he called the teacher who had failed him to say thank you (Whalen 1985).

Since many attending physicians appear reluctant to give negative feedback, the issue of how to provide negative feedback without causing interpersonal difficulties is critical. First, research on feedback recognizes the importance of credibility (Cathcart and Samovar). We are convinced that you will be perceived as credible by medical students and residents if they see that you "call 'em the way you see 'em." Do you give positive feedback when deserved as well as negative? We highly recommend the advice of Blanchard and Johnson in *The One Minute Manager* (1982): "Catch them doing something right!" In the first week of rotation, the attending physician should look for good clinical performance and give positive feedback. In this fashion, if it becomes necessary to provide negative feedback, you will have some credibility.

Second, research on feedback supports the notion that it is important to demonstrate responsiveness (Cathcart and Samovar). You will be perceived as responsive by medical students and residents if you "begin with the learner." Before providing a medical student or resident with feedback, ask for his assessment. This shows a willingness to listen. In addition, it will help if you know to whom you are talking. Is this person insightful or not? This information can help you know how careful you have to be with this person. One caution is to not let the person feel set up. So, if there are problems, provide a cue. For example, "I could see that you were having some difficulty with your case presentation this morning. I would like to talk about it, but first, would like to hear from you. How do you think it went?"

Third, research on feedback emphasizes the key role of trust. If feedback from superiors to subordinates is to have a positive impact, it is important that the receiver accurately perceive and respond to the message. Thus, the quantity of the message is less important than its relevance and accuracy (O'Reilly and Anderson 1980). There is some evidence that trust is enhanced when you "sandwich the negative feedback" between positive. According to a study of feedback to college students in a group setting, Davies and Jacobs (1985) found that the Positive-Negative-Positive Sandwich was clearly the most effective combination, with Negative-Positive-Negative the least. Also, they found that the PPN was not much better than the NNP. They concluded that, "Practically, the (PNP) 'sandwich' more than lived up to its word of mouth acclaim and should be the chosen vehicle for delivering good news and bad news in the group situation."

The PNP Sandwich is recommended by Michigan State educators in one-to-one as well as group situations, hence its moniker, "The Michigan State Sandwich." We support its use with the warning that attending physicians should not deliver a "bologna sandwich." The positive feedback has to be genuine. If bogus positive feedback is used to lead into the negative, many people will be aware of the lack of authenticity and may become defensive.

The timing of feedback is critical. In general, it should be as soon after the event as possible. However, sometimes this is not possible and may not even be desirable. It may be preferable to delay feedback if there is a need for privacy. Also, if the giver or the receiver does not have enough time to talk things over, it may be better to delay it. In addition, if either party is upset, we recommend that some time pass so that emotions can settle down. In any case, the delay should not be for more than 48 hours. Feedback should be about current performance, and, in the busy world of the hospital, things which happened more than 48 hours ago are ancient history!

The importance of feedback in clinical education was highlighted by Ende: "Without feedback, mistakes go uncorrected, good performance is not reinforced, and clinical competence is achieved empirically or not at all" (1983, p. 778). It will work best when attending physicians, residents, and medical students see themselves as allies with common goals and when the trainees solicit it themselves. The attending physician can play a key role in promoting a Total Information Learning System in which the learner sets a target and hits it.

The problems in training programs when there is not adequate feedback is typified in this diary kept by a pediatric intern, reprinted here with permission by William Morrow & Co. Do the interactions here typify your program?

Excerpts from *The Intern Blues* by Robert Marion

Sunday, August 4, 1985

Mark, a Pediatric intern, has started a new rotation in a new hospital which made his previous hospital "look like an amusement park." His resident is Rhonda, who is smart, but "treats the interns like morons."

Wednesday, August 7, 1985

Mark was on call last night and today is the "worst day of my internship." He wants to kill three people, Hanson (a four month infant who has never been out of the hospital and crumped last night), Rhonda (his second year resident) who made Mark call back the ID fellow to make sure he knew that Hanson stooled out, even though the ID fellow suggested drugs for diarrhea, and Arlene (the chief resident).

I'm going to kill Arlene. There I was sitting in the resident's room at noon today, minding my own business, trying to catch my breath; I'd made it through the night; I'd worked up six admissions. I had to keep Hanson and all the rest of them alive; I had even managed to make it through work rounds and attending rounds without falling asleep... All I wanted to do was finish my scut, write my progress notes, and get my ass out of there. But could I do that? No! Arlene came in and saw us interns sitting there, and said, "Aren't you guys going to noon conference?" Well, Elizabeth said that she had to start an IV on a kid who was supposed to go to the OR at one and Valerie said she had something else to do, and I just sat there unable to move. So Arlene said, "You know, these conferences are for you guys, not for us. It's just more work for me to schedule them. If you interns don't want to come to them, maybe we shouldn't schedule them anymore." None of us said anything back to her. I just glared. Here I was, having killed myself for over a month now. Maybe you'd think the chief resident ought to come up to us and compliment us every once in awhile, tell us we're doing a good job and that we should keep it up, but no, all we get told is that if we don't come to conferences, they're going to cut them out! So if anyone ever says anything like that to me again, I'm definitely going to kill her....

Thursday, August 8, 1985

Claire, the other chief resident, came into the residents' call room and said, "It's come to my attention that maybe we haven't been paying enough attention to you guys." That's an understatement! She told us she was sorry about it and wanted to find out what the chiefs could do to make our lives easier. And before she could say anything else, Rhonda yelled, "This makes me so damn mad! Here we are, working our rumps off. I had eleven admissions the other night and Arlene knew it but did not once did I get a 'You did a good job last night, Rhonda' or anything. All she gave me was 'If you can't get your interns to conferences, we just won't have them anymore.' You want to know what's wrong? You treat us like dirt! It wasn't so long ago that you were doing this! You can't tell me you don't remember what it's like…all you can do is complain that we're not coming to conferences. You know I'd love to able to go to the conferences. I'd like to learn something. But I don't see you or Arlene volunteering to cover the ward for me so I can go!"

I wouldn't have believed it if I hadn't seen it. Elizabeth felt that same way. Neither of us thought Rhonda had it in her to stand up for herself like that. She seems too much like a robot to show that much emotion. I mean, she's feeling as rotten about working on this ward as we are.

The rest of the exchange was pretty amazing, too. After Rhonda finished yelling, Claire said, "Rhonda, you know what we think of you. We might not always say it, but you're the best we've got. Whenever I see your name on the schedule, I breathe a sigh of relief because I know you're never going to do the wrong thing." And then Rhonda said, "You sure have a strange way of showing it. I don't expect a pat on the head just for taking night call, but I don't expect to be yelled at either."

It made me feel a little better about working with Rhonda. Who knows? Maybe I won't have to kill her after all.

Can you imagine how much better this team would have functioned if (1) Arlene and Claire, the chief residents, had given Rhonda, the second-year resident, positive feedback that when she is on call they breath a sigh of relief, and if (2) Rhonda had given Mark, Valerie, and Elizabeth, the interns, positive feedback that she knows how hard they had been working?

Assessment (so that the learning needs of medical students and residents are identified) and feedback (so that their strengths and weaknesses can be addressed) should be given a high priority because these processes are essential to efficient and effective education. A third process, evaluation, will be the focus of chapter nine. Understandably, some attending physicians do not feel comfortable evaluating medical students and residents.

Evaluation, with the word "value" imbedded in it, requires that we make judgements about another person. Even under the best of circumstances, many of us do not feel comfortable judging others. But, if there is no assessment at the start of the month and no feedback during the month, then evaluation the end of the month will be particularly problematic. The purpose of the next chapter is to help you evaluate medical students and residents when your supervision of them comes to and end.

CHAPTER 9

Evaluation of Students and Residents

Viewing clinical evaluation as a systems task...leads to this important conclusion: evaluation is, first and foremost, a management task. The process of evaluation involves information-gathering, interpreting, advising, consulting, and documenting; but the end result is a positive or negative outcome - the student either graduates or fails to graduate. This is not unlike outcomes in the management of any organization. People are hired and fired; investments are made in the development of products, and those products are released or withdrawn; and losses are acknowledged and accepted even as gains are sought (Tonesk and Buchanan 1985).

Evaluation is a systematic process of determining the extent to which instructional objectives are achieved by students (Gronlund 1968).   In the field of evaluation research, the terms *"formative"* and *"summative"* evaluation were developed in 1967 by Scriven to call attention to the different purposes of evaluation.   Formative evaluation provides information for improvement, modification, and management of programs, while summative evaluation provides information for the purpose of making judgments about the basic worth of programs. The former answers the question: "How can the program be improved?"; the latter: "Should the program be continued? If so at what level?" (Patton 1982).

Just as in program evaluation, the purpose of evaluation of students and residents is twofold. The first is to provide a "formative" evaluation. This is the daily process by which the attending will give the medical learner information that will lead to improved performance: assessment and feedback as discussed in the previous chapter. The "summative" evaluation is that which the attending must do in order to provide the medical school or the residency program with an assessment of the student's or resident's ability to function as a physician. The sum of faculty evaluations is used by medical school leadership in making decisions regarding whether students graduate and by residency program directors for credentialing physicians. In the future, this process will only become more strenuous, with hospitals and licensing agencies requiring residency directors to certify that individual physicians who trained in their programs can adequately perform specific procedures and manage specific patients problems.

Both residency programs and medical schools generally use multiple methods for evaluation of performance, including written examinations, structured clinical examinations, documentation of adequate performance of procedural skills, peer evaluations, patient record audit, and written evaluations by attendings (Blank 1984; Magarian 1990).   Program and clinical clerkship directors report that, although varying methods are used, in almost all cases, it is the subjective evaluation of the attending physicians that is most heavily weighted.

Although faculty are concerned about the subjectivity of their evaluations, evaluations through direct observation have been shown to have validity.   Carline *et al.* (1989) demonstrated that ratings by physician peers and nurses with whom the physician worked could differentiate certified and noncertified internists.   It is extremely important that ward attendings take the process of evaluation very seriously and attempt to provide the most accurate description of student performance possible.

Evaluation is difficult.   Most systems for evaluation are fraught with problems.   Faculty members are very aware of problems in evaluation systems at their institutions (Tonesk).   Among the most frequently cited problems are: 1) faculty are unwilling to record negative evaluations regarding students and residents; 2) most systems do not have a method for early warning regarding students or residents with performance problems; 3) faculty generally lack training in evaluation; 4) faculty are concerned about the methods of evaluation, including the objectivity and consistency of evaluations; 5) in most systems the guidelines for handling problem students are inadequate; 6) and finally, most program directors and supervisors of medical student clerkships complain that faculty are tardy in their submission of required evaluations.

Although there is no known remedy for the last problem, there are approaches than can help faculty to deal with these concerns. Attendings should take to heart the comment by Tonesk quoted at the beginning of this chapter, that the "summative" evaluation of students and residents is actually a management task. The process can then become more objective, easier, and clearer for everyone. Procedures that have been developed in business can be applied very effectively to medicine, for indeed, the desired outcome is the same: the production of an outstanding outcome!

John Aluise, in *Current Decisions in Child Care*, describes what he terms "the performance management system" for physicians in practice. The components of this system are parallel to the elements of the ward experience. In fact, this process is much like the "Total Information Learning System" (TILS) discussed in the previous chapter. For a practice this involves a task analysis (objectives for the ward rotation), a carefully written job description (written goals and objectives), hiring (unfortunately, attendings don't have this option!), orientation (orientation with a verbal description of the attending's expectations, and feedback from the students and residents regarding their expectations), training (teaching), and finally, a "performance appraisal system." In order for the performance appraisal system to be effective, the other parts of the system must be in place. The previous chapters have discussed these elements of ward rotations. The final task is the evaluation component.

A brief review of the essential components must be discussed in order to outline effective evaluation techniques. The first part of any evaluation is what has been said and done before. The learning objectives and expectations must have been openly discussed at the beginning of the rotation. Students and residents must know how they will be evaluated. In the TILS this is "feedforward" or "setting a target." If this step is omitted, then an accurate evaluation is not possible.

A good example of a teacher truly letting students know his expectations is a high school biology teacher who always hands to his students the test a week before it is to be given. At the first quarterly parent teacher conference, many parents were questioning the teacher and objecting to this technique. To the parents, this was inexplicable. The students could simply look up all the answers to the questions and get them right.

The teacher patiently tried to explain that the material on the test was what he wanted his students to learn, and through experience, he had found that giving students the test in advance was an a good teaching technique. The students would read the material, discuss the questions, and debate the answers for a week! If they missed a question, they were allowed to re-write their answers and re-submit them. If they then answered the question correctly, they would be given credit. The parents were incredulous. One indignant father then exclaimed, "But then how can you grade them? If they all get all the questions right, then you have to give everyone an A!" The teacher smiled, and quietly replied: "Yes, I should think that that would be every teacher's dream!" Certainly in medicine it is our goal. Every student and every resident should get A's in all aspects of patient care if they hope to provide optimal medical care.

Orientation and training follow the discussion of goals, objectives and performance standards. When all these tasks have been accomplished, it is time for the performance appraisal.

Aluise has an acronym for his performance appraisal system: PRAISE. This stands for Performance Review And Information System for Employees. These appraisals are one-to-one discussions regarding the performance of both the employee (student or resident) and the functioning of the office (the ward team and the rotation). During ward rotations, there should be at least two such encounters, one approximately midway through the rotation, so that students, residents, and attendings can use the information to improve their performance. If performance is inadequate, it is at this time that standards must be reviewed, and a remediation program begun. The second meeting occurs at the end of the rotation.

As suggested in the TILS concept of starting with the learner, Aluise suggests that the session begin with a self-appraisal: let the student or resident comment regarding what he feels is going well on the rotation, and what he is doing well. Then ask the student what areas need improvement. One method for doing this is to give students a copy of the evaluation form that the attending is expected to complete and have them evaluate themselves. Most residents will be reasonably accurate in their self-assessment. At the conclusion of the mid-rotation meeting, an agreement between students and the attending can be made about individual objectives for the remainder of the rotation.

Finally, the encounter *must be documented*. This is particularly true if there are performance problems. Documentation can consist of the form that the student completed and a form by the attending. Written comments should be included regarding both the positive and negative aspects of performance discussed and the plan for the remainder of the rotation. A copy of this should be sent to the student and to his file.

The final or end-rotation appraisal can begin with briefly reviewing the written document and discussing the progress (or lack of it) with the student. The process of the first appraisal can be repeated, with the resident or student giving a self-appraisal. The attending can then summarize the discussion and complete a final evaluation.

The process of evaluation is straightforward and enjoyable when student performance is satisfactory and has shown improvement over the course of the rotation. It is when performance is inadequate that evaluation can become a distressing experience for both attendings and learners. It is under these circumstances that an objective evaluation system such as PRAISE and TILS is most helpful.

In discussion of the "problem" student and resident, Stritham (1991) asks, "What are we to do with students and residents who don't perform to our expectations? Who don't 'get it.' What is our individual and collective responsibility to them and to their future patients?" In answering these questions, the concept of separating the behavior from the persona of the student becomes essential. This concept is demonstrated in clinical medicine by physicians who are able to handle "difficult patient encounters" rather than "difficult patients." If attendings can define the student's or resident's *encounters* as problematic, rather than labeling them as "problem students," the process of evaluation becomes more objective.

We believe that this is not just a semantic distinction. Ward attendings who can make this distinction may experience less personal stress in dealing with students who have "problematic encounters." They may also find it easier to be less judgmental and to maintain a caring and helping relationship with the person.

Although we empathize with attendings when students and residents are taxing because of their behavior or attitudes, nevertheless, as role models, it is our job as educators to do our best to remain objective, caring, and helpful.

Stitham makes the point that we assume that medical students and housestaff can take care of and help themselves:

> We throw students and interns into the pool and expect them to dog-paddle in July, sidestroke in September, do the crawl in December, and butterfly in April. Those who are still dog-paddling in November or who have to be fished out of the pool too many times cannot be assimilated. The "system" throws up its collective hands, refers the individuals to the advancement committee, and says, "It's OK because they're going into psychiatry or orthopedics" (or whatever service they're not on at the moment). We assume that the next rotation will take care of the problem.

The ward attending is a part of a system that has to function effectively if problem students are going to be identified and either prescribed a remedial program that will address the problems or dismissed from school or the residency program. Identification through evaluation is the responsibility of the clinical attendings. The school or the residency program is then responsible for designing an overall remediation program.

Too often, attendings will be frustrated when systems do not seem to be responsive. One of the frequently heard reasons for not giving negative evaluations when they are warranted is that "nothing is done anyway." Even when this is true, however, it does not relieve the attending from the obligation of providing accurate evaluation of students and residents, although it seems to be a difficult and painful process.

Use of a management model for evaluation facilitates the assessment and evaluation of students with performance problems because the procedures are defined and objective. Using Aluise's performance appraisal system, the first step is to ascertain whether, in fact, there is a problem with performance. Often failures of communication lead to conflicts or mistakes that can be interpreted as inadequacy on the part of a student or resident. One example is the student who is very quiet or self-conscious, who has difficulty speaking up during rounds. Assessment of this student's knowledge base can be difficult. Others, through lack of experience, may need help understanding their role.

A student may not have known whom to call during the night when he needed help, or might have been afraid to call a resident who has previously complained about his "dependency" or "stupid questions." Some may simply lack the knowledge or experience to handle a specific problem, indicating that they need further training.

In analyzing the etiology of a problem with other staff and with the student or resident, the attending must do so in as objective a manner as possible. Essentially there are three main categories to examine in most cases: the tasks performed, the timeliness in which tasks are done, and finally, the relationship between the problem student or resident and others involved. If, after investigation and observation of the student or resident, it is obvious that there is a skill deficiency, a remediation program should be planned. An example would be having a resident repeat an Advance Life Support course if he had not performed well during a cardiac arrest.

If the issue is not a deficiency in skills, or if the deficiency has been addressed and the student's or resident's performance is still deemed inadequate, then it is likely that the issue is related to attitude. If, consistently, tasks are not performed in a timely manner, or if the student or resident seems to have repeated conflicts with others, it is necessary to objectively observe, describe, and document the behavior. The student or resident then should be confronted either in a one-to-one session with the attending, or, in some cases, with the attending and another appropriate supervisor, e.g. the supervisory resident, the nursing supervisor.

Again, start with the learner and ask for a self-assessment. This is most appropriately done by asking if the student or resident is aware of the problem. Unfortunately it is usually the students with inappropriate attitudes who have little insight. Many will blame their performance on others.

If the student or resident does not perceive his difficulties, he should be presented with an objective assessment: This is the behavior that we see. Describe the behavior in objective terms, just as in the example given on communication through the medical chart: don't write, the patient was drunk, say instead that the patient was unsteady, smelled of alcohol, and admitted to drinking a pint of whiskey.

In his article "Educational Malpractice," Stitham wrote an excellent description of a problem student, starting first with some rather subjective descriptions, but going on to objective descriptions of behaviors that support his subjective assessment:

> He was the worst student I had ever encountered. His affect tended toward the surly; he had trouble expressing himself and substantial difficulty in putting the picture together. Even at the end of four weeks, he would still list "bronchoscopy" as the problem, not as part of the plan. He left his stethoscope in his ears when we discussed a patient's examination at the bedside. He didn't make eye contact with anyone. He was eager to leave the hospital at precisely 5 PM (Stitham 1991).

Outline the issues clearly and precisely with the problem learner. Be candid about the limits that will be set regarding the expected performance standards, and what the consequences will be if the standards are not met within a specified period of time. Depending upon the problem, consequences may be as severe as probation or dismissal from a program. Opportunities for learning and improving behavior must be made available to the student.

We cannot overemphasize that it is essential to *document in writing* the problems encountered. A clear description should be written regarding the objective behaviors observed, the discussion with the student, the expected standards, the remediation plan for this rotation, and the time when the problem will be reassessed. While confidentiality must be respected, this documentation should be forwarded to the appropriate faculty, such as the clerkship director, the program director, and the student's or resident's advisor.

After the process has begun, it is the responsibility and choice of the student or resident to conform to standards. At the end of the specified time period, the attending and the other supervisory personnel should reevaluate the problem. If no progress has been made, then the consequences that have been previously agreed to would be enforced.

The ward attending should work with the program director and/or clerkship director when there are performance problems, for the overall evaluation of students and residents remains his responsibility. If there are problems with performance, the attending should plan and assist in implementing a remediation program for the student for that rotation. The long-term planning for continued performance evaluation and remediation remain the responsibility of the medical school and program directors.

Although faculty are reportedly hesitant to write negative reports, it is essential that deficiencies in performance be documented and addressed. Failure to do so means that we will produce incompetent physicians. All too often, program directors are aware that there are "problem residents" but have no data to support the alleged inadequacies, and therefore no method for designing a remediation plan.

The end result is a positive or negative outcome. The student or resident either graduates or fails to graduate. It is the process of evaluation that allows this distinction to be made. Attendings are obligated to provide objective evaluations in order to ensure that we do not endorse incompetency. Only in this manner can we protect the welfare of patients.

In the epilogue, Dr. Clifford Straehley, recently retired, provides us with a long term perspective of the responsibilities of attendings.

Epilogue

*Responsibilities of the Teaching Staff
in Medical Education*

By Clifford Straehley, M.D.

The major responsibility of a training Program Director in all fields of medicine is to assure an excellent learning environment for residents and their adequate supervision by a dedicated and capable attending staff. Another responsibility is to mount an effective quality assurance program to shield residents, in so far as possible, from malpractice litigation because they no longer enjoy relative immunity from such actions in today's litigious climate.   These considerations raise two questions:

1. Should a clinical department in teaching hospital define explicitly the responsibilities of its teaching staff?

2.   Should there be in force some mechanism for assessing the effectiveness of the attending staff/faculty as teachers?

The Surgical Department at the University of Hawaii John A. Burns School of Medicine was urged by its legal counsel to prepare a memorandum of understanding (Appendix A) to define the responsibilities of the surgical teaching staff. It was the intent of the Department Chairman that all regular and clinical faculty members, upon familiarizing themselves with the content of the memorandum, would sign an agreement binding themselves to abide by its terms.

The stimulus for this effort grew out of a difficult and regrettable event which occurred when a participating teaching hospital and the University of Hawaii, John A. Burns School of Medicine Integrated Residency Training Program in Surgery, were named as defendants in a malpractice action in which the attending surgeon had been excused by the plaintiff. During ensuing litigation the attending surgeon became an adversary of the residency program and the hospital.

Because we were unable to find a published report of an issue such as this, we circulated our newly developed memorandum together with a questionnaire pertaining to the issues raised by it to the program directors of all approved general surgical training programs in the United States. The questionnaire was designed to sample opinions regarding what responsibilities attending surgeons and/or faculty members owe to surgical residents as well as to the training program of which they are a part. What is the bond between the attending surgeon and the resident and what obligation does the former owe to the latter? There were 214 responses for 282 programs (76 percent).

Of the responding programs, 68 (31.7 percent) already had a written document defining the responsibilities of the attending staff/faculty and 21 of these programs require that all attending surgeons who participate with residents in direct patient care sign the document. There were 146 responding programs which do not presently use such a document and of these 57 (39 percent) are considering doing so in the future. It is of interest to note that 43 percent of non-university affiliated training programs negotiate a written memorandum of understanding with attending staff whereas only 25 percent of university sponsored programs do so.

Opinions concerning the usefulness of such a document varied widely and the majority of programs appended written commentary a sampling of which follows:

I think it is an excellent memorandum and I am considering using something similar.

I rely more on the goodwill of the Attending Staff rather that the language of a document.

I guess I do not understand why such a document is necessary, or what such a document is supposed to accomplish.

Excellent. This delineates in print an understanding which exists in our program. It documents the concept of responsibility for surgical education and is not in anyway way perceivable as being threatening.

Basically I think it is an excellent idea which will probably be mandated by our legal system within the next few years. I intend to present it to our faculty.

I believe these are generally accepted "points of behavior." I am uncertain what real purpose these serve.

It's well put and could serve as a national standard. While it may satisfy legal concerns and may be necessary for multihospital program it is not so critical in a close knit staff. The proper philosophy must emanate from the leader and its acceptance reflects the degree to which the staff has been adequately educated.

A fine document - we have gone one step further by having faculty annually complete a Management-by-Agreement Form.

My reaction is negative. Majority of attending surgeons go into teaching because they enjoy and like it. They do not need to sign a document to remind them they are there to teach. It is the responsibility of the Program Director to ensure the teaching faculty are doing their job.

Twelve university programs and seven non-university affiliated programs indicated in their comments a concern that the memorandum raised legal issues.

The following comments reflect their concerns:

Are you developing or avoiding a medical-legal trap with this document?

A sad state of affairs when you must resort to the "law" for direction of the Surgical Staff, however, I understand the necessity.

I would not think this sort of memo necessary. I believe they go without saying even in this bureaucratic and litigious age.

Legal counsel gone wild.

More paperwork. Now I'm sure we will have to do something similar to satisfy lawyers.

If I can read between the lines, it is a reaction to litigation and not an effort to improve resident education.

Interesting document: its ability to hold up in court, of course, must be taken. I'm not sure it provides a coverage but it does remind attendings of their responsibility to patients, residents, and teaching.

I think that your document, if discovered by a plaintiff's attorney, would place your program and your attending staff in a poor liability exposure situation.

It may have legal value protecting the hospital/ department but should be superfluous for full-time faculty . . . .

Queried specifically about the responsibility of each surgical faculty member or attending surgeon to assess the level of capability of each surgical resident with whom he works, 100 percent of the responding program directors agreed that this important responsibility was incumbent upon surgical faculty and attendings. With only two exceptions, virtually all respondents (99 percent) agreed that ultimate responsibility for the welfare of the patient lies with the attending surgeon. Perhaps this attitude was expressed best by one respondent who stated: "The attending surgeon is legally, morally and ethically responsible for each patient.

Residents do not legally have Hospital Privileges nor do I believe they should." Regarding the proposition that resident surgeons are "learners" and cannot function without supervision by attending staff/faculty, there was considerable diversity of opinion. While 82 percent of the program directors agreed, others expressed different concerns:

Trying to define exactly how much or little supervision is necessary is impossible, for each individual resident and each type of case demands varying degrees of supervision.

The staff cannot be present at all times and the Residency Review Committee also states the resident must have opportunity for independent action.

Our hospital receives a large volume of trauma and it is imperative that the resident participate in the initial resuscitation and sometimes take the patient to the operating room while waiting for the private attending to arrive.

I feel supervision may be direct or indirect depending on experience and competence of the resident and the task to be performed.

The concept of the "teaching resident" would be adversely affected if the statement were taken as all or none. A competent senior resident may supplant attending supervision without negative patient care consequences.

It seems probable that this diversity of opinion arose because of an inherent ambiguity in what constitutes "supervision" of a resident surgeon by attending staff. Clearly a resident who has benefitted from close personal supervision and an excellent learning experience over time and has demonstrated consistent

competence should be permitted to act independently in
crisis situations. This concept however does not imply
that the attending surgeon is relieved of responsibility for
the outcome of actions so delegated.

We were surprised to learn that 32 programs (15
percent) had encountered a situation such as ours in
which a malpractice action was filed against a resident
surgeon and the attending surgeon was not named as a
co-defendant. Comments appended to this particular
question indicate that the episode for some had proved to
be disruptive. The responses from these programs
underscore how inconsistent and arbitrary malpractice
litigation has become in the United States:

*Generally doesn't happen (here). Residents are usually
released from suits relatively rapidly.*

*Many attendings and chief of surgery were deposed as
were several of the residents. The suit was against the hospital
and the resident. It is anticipated when this suit is settled, that
the attending will then be sued.*

*. . . When the suit was filed the attending's insurance
settled out of court early for a small sum and the institution
with a "deep pocket" insuring the resident was sued for a large
sum.*

There is a strongly expressed opinion among program directors that resident surgeons should not be
abandoned to stand alone in malpractice actions:

*We "join" all resident suits if the resident was acting
within the scope of his/her responsibilities.*

Residents are agents of the hospital . . . the hospital should answer their defense.

We got the resident dropped from the suit. The suit was changed to include the staff.

An exception to this concept was forcefully stated by one respondent:

The attending surgeon cannot and must not be held responsible for every action of the resident. When the resident commits an act of willful misconduct or gross negligence he can be held accountable on his own.

In the event of a malpractice action should the attending surgeon be held responsible for the patient outcome? One program director stated what seems to be the prevailing opinion tersely and with force:

All of our attending surgeons are held responsible for direct patient care. Resident surgeons are not credentialled to practice surgery.

If, for whatever reason, the attending surgeon does not participate in the defense of a malpractice action, it can prove to be very disruptive for the program and affect morale:

It is a serious concern.

All attempts to change the defendant were unsuccessful.

We defended the case, but the attending private surgeon sought to blame the resident for the " ? malpractice".

We fought it and won. The fault lay with the surgeon but the patient directed it toward the resident.

The situation was an extremely difficult one in which the resident and attending had to have separate defense, and the attending maintained that the resident should be solely at fault.

Today the directors of training programs must concern themselves not only with the educational and training issues that enable their programs to fulfill the rigorous requirements of the Residency Review Committees but also with legal and ethical questions that could risk liability. Barton (1991) has even directed attention to the unpleasant reality that "the subject of malpractice insurance should be of concern to every resident." She stresses the fact that courts "seem to focus on the issue of supervision and control" of the resident's activities.

Indeed a recent communication by Shulkin (1990) stresses that physician training programs are no longer regarded as "protected environments" by the courts. Extrapolating from a 1984 U.S. General Accounting Office study, Shulkin estimated that 1800 residents would have been named in legal suits during that year. He cited a study of medical malpractice litigation involving residents published by the Risk Management Foundation of the Harvard Medical Institutions Forum (1989). This report found that residents in surgical specialties were the most vulnerable of all trainees.

A considerable body of legal literature provides case studies in which residents and training programs have been named as defendants in malpractice actions.

Hospitals and attending surgeons have been named as co-defendants often under the doctrine of "respondent superior;" however, unequivocal instances in which the attending surgeon was excused as a defendant in an action against a resident or the training program are not documented. Although there is a handful of papers that address the legal liability of medical students and residents in training, a search of the medical literature did not disclose a discussion of specific examples of the failure of an attending surgeon to stand with a resident in defense of a malpractice action.

Kapp (1983) published a thoughtful analysis of these issues which could be read profitably by the program directors of all training programs. He has made very concrete recommendations as a result of his analysis of "the real potential for legal liability, direct or vicarious, flowing from patient care rendered by medical trainees." His first recommendation is that "every medical school clinical department should draft and enforce written guidelines concerning supervisory expectations of faculty members. These should be explicitly accepted by each faculty member as a condition of faculty appointment . . . "We have sought for reasons why only 31.7 percent of programs responding to this survey currently have written memorandums of understanding with attending surgeons and faculty. A substantial number of university program directors stated that a separate document is unnecessary because the responsibilities of their faculty members are clearly delineated in the faculty contract. Other program directors feel that the time tested traditional and ideals of the surgical educator implicitly define the obligations of the teacher of surgery to the resident surgeon which makes a written document irrelevant. Such idealism was expressed in statements such as:

We have taken these espoused principles for granted.

I believe these are generally accepted points of behavior.

The responsibility of surgeons to cooperate is not vested in a written document.

We have always relied on good faith.

Several program directors indicated that they viewed our faculty memorandum of understanding as an acceptable, precise and appropriate general statement, but hastened to point out that a written document does not ensure scrupulous compliance with imposed responsibilities. They asked how a deficient attending surgeon is to be removed from his position on the teaching staff?

One respondent wrote: "It is well written and pertinent to the issue; its greatest usefulness may be in ruling out those attendings who exploit residents and provide marginal teaching."

There was virtually unanimous agreement that attending surgeons must evaluate carefully the capability of each surgical resident to manage adequately all tasks delegated by the staff member to the resident and that the ultimate responsibility for the welfare of the patient lies with the attending surgeon.

In the event of malpractice litigation directed at the resident surgeon those program directors who made specific comments indicated a strongly held opinion that the training program and the attending surgeon should support the resident throughout the action unless there had been "willful misconduct or gross negligence."

One-hundred and seventy three program directors wrote specific comments characterizing their reaction to the memorandum of understanding that we have developed at the University of Hawaii.   One-hundred and twenty (69.4 percent) of these were judged to be favorable, 34 (19.6 percent) indifferent and 19 (11 percent) unfavorable.   Unfavorable comments seemed to arise from philosophical and emotional objections to the idea that present day contingency might require an explicit memorandum of understanding with faculty and attending surgeons.   Barton states that these "comments reflect[ed] a dangerous naivete and a defensive attitude toward the legal system."   She adds that "I have always been concerned about an approach that informally recognized specific legal responsibilities but is unwilling to acknowledge publicly those same responsibilities for fear that they will become more onerous." It is true that traditions dating from Hippocrates and the Pythagoreans should have forged a covenantal bond between teachers and students (1967). Issues defining the distinctions between a contract and a covenantal bond have been brilliantly explored by May in his monograph entitled *The Physician's Covenant - Images of the Healer in Medical Ethics*. A contract of course is a legal document. If a signatory breaches a contract he or she may be exposed to legal action. On the other hand, a covenantal bond imposes a moral obligation but no legal restraint.

The forces that compel adherence to the injunctions of an unwritten covenantal bond are tradition (often religious or spiritual), a sense of community, honor, personal integrity, a sense of duty, obligation, and deeply felt sense of indebtedness. These forces are attributes of character. As May states "confidence (is) put in their reliability without any insistency on formal guarantees." Unfortunately, in this less than perfect world and in a litigious age, prudent administrators will be well advised to supplement the spiritual force of a covenant with the legal force of a contract. As Barton forcefully maintains administrators should "prefer a proactive approach that is willing to acknowledge publicly [legal] responsibilities . . . and respond to situations in a manner that indicates the exercise of judgement in light of the responsibilities rather that in ignorance of them."

After careful consideration of the issues involved, I conclude that all program directors of training programs in surgery or other medical specialties should develop a memorandum of understanding with their faculty and that all staff who have attending or teaching responsibilities should sign the document.

It follows that the failure of a faculty member to comply with the requirements of the document would afford grounds for dismissal for the faculty. The chairman and executive committee of a teaching department should establish a valid mechanism for assessing the effectiveness of attending staff as teachers. It must be stressed that, while service is important, the primary purpose of a training program is educational. To be a teacher is not a birthright. It is a privilege which is earned.

Appendix A

Responsibilities of the Surgical Teaching Staff
University of Hawaii Department of Surgery
Integrated Residency Training Program

As a member of the Surgical Department teaching faculty, you will play a major role in instructing residents in the principles and practice of surgery and its applicable surgical basic sciences. The most effective surgical teaching occurs during patient encounters in the office or clinical setting, at the bedside, or in the operating room. Frequent, close interaction between resident staff, their attending surgeons and the patients under their care are necessary for the successful teaching of surgery.

Your acceptance of an appointment on the teaching surgical faculty indicates your willingness to assume the following responsibilities toward the surgical residency training programs:

1. Accept the responsibility for the surgical resident(s) assigned to your patients.

2. Allow the resident(s) to actively participate under your supervision and control in the care of your patients, including the performance of procedures, commensurate with the residents' level of training.

3. Willingness to discuss your patients' problems in detail with the resident(s) assigned to the case or other residents if they ask

4. Willingness to participate in teaching conferences with the resident staff when requested to do so.

5. Willingness to participate in the annual or more frequent evaluations of the resident staff when asked by the Program Director or Directors of Surgical Education.

6. Attend regularly scheduled University Surgical Department Rounds and other special teaching conferences such as visiting professor lectures and mobidity-mortality conferences.

7. Share your knowledge and information about surgery with the residents including discussion of resident's cases and problems.

8. Provide follow-up information concerning patients for whom you and your resident have cared so that the resident may have a fuller awareness of the outcome of surgical management.

9. Maintenance of surgical privileges and active participation in the surgical staff affairs of at least one teaching hospital in the Integrated Surgical Residency Training Program.

10. Make reasonable effort to keep current with advances in surgical knowledge and participate in continuing medical education.

11. Serve on hospital committees which relate to peer review and quality of care when asked to do so.

It is desirable that all surgical faculty members should be aware of the fact that surgical residents are learners in a program designed to help them master to the fullest extent of their capability the art and science of surgery. Residents have not reached that point in their careers when they can function without supervision by the surgical faculty member to assess the level of capability of each surgical resident with whom he works. All responsibilities which a surgical resident assumes are thus delegated responsibilities. Ultimately the attending surgeon is the one responsible for the welfare of the patients under his care and of the residents' participation in the management of those patients.

REFERENCES

AAMC. "Panel Report on the General Education of the Physician: Physicians for the Twenty-First Century." *Journal of Medical Education* 59(11): 1984.

Aliuse, John. *Current Decisions in Infant and Child Care.* Little Falls: Health Learning Systems Inc., 1990.

Anderson, Scarvia B. *et al. Encyclopedia of Educational Evaluation.* San Francisco: Jossey-Bass Publishers, 1977.

Association of American Medical Colleges. *Journal of Medical Education.* 59(11): 1984.

Atkins, Stuart. *The Name of Your Game.* Beverly Hills: Ellis and Stewart, 1981.

Auden, W. H. and Kronenberger, Louis. *The Viking Book of Aphorisms.* New York: Penguin Books, 1981.

Barton, E. L. "Personal Communication."

Barton, E. L. "What Residents Should Know About Malpractice Insurance." *Minnesota Physician,* Feb. 1991.

Berquist, William H. and Phillips, Steven R. *A Handbook for Faculty Development*. Washington, D.C.: Council for the Advancement of Small Colleges, 1975.

Betcher, R. William. *A Student to Student Guide to Medical School: Study Strategies, Mneumonics, Personal Growth*. New York: Little Brown and Company, 1985.

Bishop, F. Marian. "Preceptorships in the Twenty-First Century." *Utah Medical Association Bulletin* 35(6): 12, 14, 1987.

Blank LL, Grosso LJ, and Benson JA. "A Survey of Clinical Skills Evaluaton Practice in Internal Medicine Residency Programs." *Journal of Medical Education* 59: 401-406, 1984.

Bloom, Benjamin *et al. Taxonomy of Educational Objectives: Handbook I. Cognitive Domain*. New York: McKay, 1956.

Bradford, Leland P. "The Teaching-Learning Transaction." *Adult Education* 8(3): 135-145, 1958.

Bruffee, Kenneth. "Collaborative Learning and 'The Conversation of Mankind' "*College English* 46(6): 635-652, 1984.

Bursztajn, Harold *et al. Medical Choices, Medical Chances: How Patients, Families, and Physicians Cope with Uncercainty*. New York: Delacore Press, 1981.

Cantor, Joel C. *et al.* "Medical Educators' Views on Medical Education Reform." *Journal of the American Medical Association* 265(8): 1001-1006, 1991.

Capobianco AT. *The Development of a System for Evaluation. National League for Nursing.* New York: Publication Number 23-1775, 1979.

Carter WB, Inui TS, Kukull WA, Haigh VH. "Outcome-Based Doctor-Patient Interaction Analysis: II. Identifying Effective Provider and Patient Behavior." *Medical Care.* 20:550-556, 1982.

Cathart, Robert S. and Samovar, Larry A. *Small Group Communication.* Dubuque: Wm. C. Brown Publishers, 1989.

Collins, George F., Cassie, Josephine M., and Daggett, Christopher J. "The Role of the Attending Physician in Clinical Training." *The Journal of Medical Education* 53: 429-431, 1978.

Daly, James J. and Tysinger, James W. "Microbiology Clinical Conferences: Expanding the Roles and Responsibilties of Faculty and Students." *Teaching and Learning in Medicine* 1(4): 211-214, 1989.

Davies, D. and Jacobs, A. " 'Sandwiching' Complex Interpersonal Feedback." *Small Group Behavior* 16: 387-396, 1985.

Dodge, W.T. "Communication and Interpersonal Skills."
    In *Fundamentals of Family Medicine,* edited by
    Robert B. Taylor. New York: Springer-Verlag,
    1983.

Donnelly WJ. "Medical Language as Symptom: Doctor
    Talk in Teaching Hospitals." *Perspectives in Biology
    and Medicine* 30: 81-94, 1986.

Duffy LD, Hamerman D and Cohen MA.
    "Communicaton Skills of House Officers: A Study
    in a Medical Clinic." *Annals of Internal Medicine*
    93:354-357, 1980.

Eble, Kenneth. *The Craft of Teaching.* San Francisco:
    Jossey-Bass Publishers, 1988.

Edelstein, L. "Ancient Medicine. The Hippocratic Oath:
    Text, Translation and Interpretation. Selected
    Papers of Ludwig Edelstein." Eds. Temkin, O. and
    Temkin. C.L. Baltimore, The Johns Hopkins
    University Press, 1967.

Edwards JC and Brannan JR. "Case Presentation Format
    and Clinical Reasoning: A Stragegy for Teaching
    Medical Students." *Medical Teaching* 9: 285-292,
    1987.

Ende, Jack. "Feedback in Clinical Medical Education."
    Journal of the American Medical Association 250(6):
    777-781, 1983.

Engel, George L. "What If Music Students Were Taught To Play Their Instruments as Medical Students Are Taught To Interview." *Pharos* Fall: 12-13, 1982.

Ficklin, Fred L. *et al.* "Faculty and Housestaff Members as Role Models." *Journal of Medical Education* 63(5): 392-396, 1988.

Freidenheim, Milt. "Removing the Warehouse from Cost-Conscious Hospitals." *The New York Times:* F5, March 3, 1991.

Gibb, Jack R. "Is Help Helpful?" *Forum*: 25-27, February, 1964.

Gil, Doron H., Heins, Marilyn, and Jones, Patricia B. "Perceptions of Medical School Faculty Members and Students on Clinical Clerkship Feedback." *Journal of Medical Education* 59(11): 856-864, 1984.

Gronlund NE. *Constructing Achievement Tests. 3rd ed.* New York: MacMillan Publishing Company 1976.

Hampton JR, Harrison MJG, Mitchell JRA, Prichard JS, Seymour C. "Relative Contributions of History Taking, Physical Examination, and Laboratory Investigation to Diagnosis and Management of Medical Outpatients." *British Medical Journal* 2: 486-9, 1975.

Hanson, Phillip G. "Giving Feedback: An Interpersonal Skill." *The 1975 Annual Handbook for Group Facilitators*. LaJolla: University Associates Publishers, Inc., 1975.

Harden RM. "Assess Students: An Overview." *Medical Teacher* 1: 65-70,1979.

Healy, Charles C. and Welchert, Alice J. "Mentoring Relations: A Definition to Advance Research and Practice." *Educational Researcher:* December, 1990, 17-21.

Huffman EK. *Medical Record Management.* Berwn, Illinois: Physicians' Record Company, p.123, 1972.

Irby, David M. "Clinical Teaching and the Clinical Teacher." *Journal of Medical Education* 61(9) Part 2: 35-45, 1986.

Iserson KV. "The Supervision of Physicians in Training: An Educational and Ethical Dilemma." *Medical Teacher* 10:195-201, 1988.

Kapp, M.B. "Legal Implications of Clinical Supervision of Medical Students and Residents. *Journal of Medical Education* 58:293-99, 1983.

Kassirer, Jerome P. and Kopelman, Richard I. *Learning Clinical Reasoning.* Baltimore: Williams and Wilkins, 1991.

King, Thomas C. "Encouraging Residents to Learn." In *Surgical Teaching: Practice Makes Perfect* by Neal Whitman and Peter Lawrence. Salt Lake City: University of Utah School of Medicine, 1991.

Langsley DG. "Medical Competence and Performance Assessment: A New Era." *Journal of American Medical Association* 266:977-980, 1991.

Levinson, Daniel. *The Seasons of a Man's Life.* New York: Alfred A. Knopf, 1978.

Lichstein PR and Nieman LZ: "Diagnosing Technique Problems in Interviewing Patients." *Journal of Medical Education* 60:566-568, 1985.

Lipkin M, Quill TE, Napodano RJ. "The Medical Interview: A Core Curriculum for Residencies in Internal Medicine." *Annals of Internal Medicine* 100:277-284, 1984.

Lobeck, Charles C. and Stone, Howard L. "Class Mentors: A Step Toward Implementing the GPEP Report." *Academic Medicine* 65(6): 351-354, 1990.

Lutz L, Schultz D, and Litton EM. "Diagnosis Formulation by Residents and Physicians at Different Levels of Experience." *Journal of Medical Education* 61:984-987, 1986.

Magarian GJ and Mazure DJ. "Evaluation of Students in Medicine Clerkships." *Academic Medicine* 65: 341-345, 1990.

Mageean RJ. "Study of 'Discharge Communications' from Hospital." *British Medical Journal* 293: 1283-1284, 1986.

May, W.F. "The Physician's Covenant. Images of the Healer in Medical Ethics."

McDonough, WJ. "Residents in Medical Malpractice: A Review of Claims History." Risk Management Foundation of Harvard Medical Institutions, Inc. Forum, May-June 1989.

McLagan, Patricia A. *Helping Others Learn*. Reading, MA: Addison-Wesley Publishing Company, 1978.

McLeod PJ. " Assessing the Value of Student Case Write-ups and Write-up Evaluations." *Academic Medicine* 64:273-274, 1989.

Miller, George. "The Background to Modern Psychology." In G. Miller, editor. *States of Mind*. New York: Pantheon Books, 1983.

Miller, Lewis H. "Hubris in the Academy: Can Teaching Survive an Overwhelming Quest for Excellence." *Change* : 9-11, 53, September-October, 1990.

Mir MA, Marshall RJ, Evans RW, Hall R, and Duthie HL. "Comparision between Videotape and Personal Teaching as Methods of Communicating Clinical Skills to Medical Students." *British Medical Journal* 289 (6436): 31-34, 1984.

Moran MT, Wiser TH, Nanda J, and Gross H. "Measuring Medical Residents' Chart Documentation Practices." *Journal of Medical Education* 63: 859-865, 1988.

Morgan MK and Irby DM. *Evaluating Clinical Competence in the Health Professions.* Saint Louis: The C.V. Mosby Company, 1978.

Morrison S. "The Ideal Chart." *Maryland Medical Journal* 35:261, 1986.

NaPier PM and NaPier BL. "Medical charts and malpractice: How to avoid costly errors and omissions." *Hawaii Medical Journal* 48:596-597, 600, 607, 1989.

Neame, R.L.B. and Powis, D.A. "Toward Independent Learning: Curriculum Design for Assisting Students: To Learn How to Learn." *Journal of Medical Education* 56(11): 886-893, 1981.

Office of Medical Education Research and Development. "Characteristics of Constructive Feedback in Medical Education." East Lansing: Michigan State University, undated handout.

Palmer, Parker J. "Good Teaching: A Matter of Living the Mystery."*Change* 22(1): 10-16, 1990.

Patton MQ. *Creative Evaluation.* Newbury Park: Sage Publications, 2nd ed., 1987.

Patton MQ. *Practical Evaluation.* Newbury Park: Sage Publications, 1982.

Penney TM. "How to do it: Dictate a Discharge Summary." *British Medical Journal* 298:1084-5, 1989.

Pfeiffer, J. William and Jones, John E. "Openness, Collusion and Feedback." *The 1972 Annual Handbook for Group Facilitators*. LaJolla: University Associates Publishers, Inc., 1972.

Platt FW, McMath JC. "Clinical Hypocompetence: the Interview." *Annals of Internal Medicine*. 91:898-902, 1979.

Poirier S and Brauner DJ. "Ethics and the Daily Language of Medical Discourse." *Hastings Center Report* . 5-9, 1988.

Prater, Marsha. "Teaching Procedures" in *Surgical Teaching: Practice Makes Perfect* by Neal Whitman and Peter Lawrence. Salt Lake City: University of Utah School of Medicine, 1991.

Prather H. *Notes to Myself*. Moab, Utah: Real People Press, 1970.

Quirk M and Letendre A. "Teaching Communication Skills to First-Year Medical Students." *Journal of Medical Education* 61: 603-605, 1986.

Raskova, Jana, Martin, Eugene C., and Shea, Stephen, M. "A Second-Year Pathology Course that Emphasizes Independent Learning." *Journal of Medical Education* 63(6): 486-488, 1988.

Ratner, Joseph, editor. *Intellegence in the Modern World: John Dewey's Philosophy.* New York: Random House, 1939.

Reilly DE. *Behavioral Objectives in Nursing: Evaluation of Learner Attainment.* New York: Appleton-Century-Crofts, 1975.

Romm FJ and Putnam SM. "The Validity of the Medical Record." *Medical Care* 19: 310-315, 1981.

Rossi PH and Freeman HE. *Evaluation: A Systmatic Approach.* Newbury Park: Sage Publications, 4th ed., 1989.

Russell, John. *The New York Times*: H33, April 16, 1989.

Sadler, D. "Education and Improvement of Academic Learning." *Journal of Higher Education* 54(1): 60-79, 1983.

Sanders PS, Chairperson, MMIE Risk Management Committee. "Risk Management in Practice: Maintaining Defensible Medical Records (Part Three)." *Minnesota Medicine* 70: 591, 1987.

Sanders PS, Chairperson, MMIE Risk Management Committee. "Risk Management in Practice: Maintaining Defensible Medical Records." *Minnesota Medicine* 70: 471, 473, 1987.

Sanders PS, Chairperson, MMIE Risk Management Committee. "Risk Management in Practice: Maintaining Defensible Medical Records (Part Two)." *Minnesota Medicine* 70: 535, 1987.

Sapira, Joseph D. "A Modest Proposal: Board Certifictation for Medical Educators (or Quis Custodiet Ipsos Custodes?)" *Southern Medical Journal* 79(9): 1141-1142, 1986.

Schwenk, Thomas L. and Whitman, Neal. *Residents as Teachers*. Salt Lake City: University of Utah School of Medicine, 1984.

Schwenk, Thomas L. and Whitman, Neal. *The Physician as Teacher*. Baltimore: Williams and Wilkins, 1987.

Scriven M. "The Methodology of Evaluation." R. Tyler, R. Gagne, and M. Scriven (Eds.), *Perspectives on curriculum evaluation*. AERA Monograph Series on Curriculum Evaluation, No. 1. Chicago: Rand McNally, 1967.

Seldin, Peter. "Evaluating Teaching Performance: Answers to Common Questions." *AAHE Bulletin* 40: 10, 1987.

Seldin, Peter. "What Does It Take to Change Campus Cultures?" *Academic Leader* 7(4): 1, 1991.

Sheehan, T. Joseph. "Feedback: Giving and Receiving." *Journal of Medical Education* 59(11): 913, 1984.

Shulkin, DJ. "Resident Forum - Potential Liability Problems." *Journal of American Medical Association* 264 (1) : 24, 1990.

Siegler, Mark *et al.* "Effect of Role-Model Clinicians on Students' Attitudes in a Second Year Course on Introduction to the Patient." *Journal of Medical Education* 62(11): 935-937, 1987.

Smith, Lloyd. "Medical Education for the 21st Century." *Journal of Medical Education* 60(2): 106-112, 1985.

Stitham S. "Educational malpractice." *Journal of American Medical Association* 266: 905-906, 1991.

Stritter, Frank. "A Developmental Approach to Clinical Instruction." *Family Practice Faculty Development Center of Texas Newsletter* 7(1): 1-5, 1986.

Stritter, Frank, Hain, Jack, and Grimes, David A. "Clinical Teaching Reexamined." *Journal of Medical Education* 50: 876-882, 1975.

Struening EL and Guttentag M. *Handbook of Evaluation Research.* Beverly Hills: Sage Publications, 1975.

Thomas, Lewis. "The Art of Teaching Science." *The New York Times Magazine:* March 14, 1982.

Tiberius, Richard G. "The Influence of Student Evaluative Feedback on the Improvement of Clinical Teaching."*Journal of Higher Education* 60 (6): 665-681, 1989.

Tonesk X. and Buchanan R. "Faculty Perceptions of Current Clincial Evaluation Systems." *Journal of Medical Education* 60: 573-576, 1985.

Tosti D. "Formative Feedback." *NSPI Journal* 17(8): 19-21, 1978.

Tulloch AJ, Fowler GH, McMullan JJ, and Spence JM. Hospital Discharge Reports: Content and Design. *British Medical Journal* 4: 443-446, 1975.

Verrier, David and Leser, Anne. *Teaching in the Clinical Setting: A Handbook*. Columbus: The Ohio State University, 1990.

Weed LL. Medical Records that Guide and Teach. *New England Journal of Medicine* 278: 593-599, 652-657, 1968.

Weiner, Norbert. *Cybernetics and Society*. Boston: Houghton Mifflin Co., 1950.

Whalen, James P. "Evaluating Students." *Journal of Medical Education* 60(7): 584, 1985.

White KB, Beary JF. "Illegible Handwritten Medical Records." *New England Journal of Medicine* 314: 390-91, 1986.

Whitman, Neal. "A Total Information Learning System." *Focus on Surgical Education* 2(4): 14-15, 1985.

Whitman, Neal. *Creative Medical Teaching*. Salt Lake City: University of Utah School of Medicine, 1988.

Whitman, Neal and Lawrence, Peter. *Surgical Teaching: Practice Makes Perfect*. Salt Lake City: University of Utah School of Medicine, 1991.

Whitman, Neal and Roth, Craig. "Evaluations Teaching Improvement Strategies." *Journal of Staff, Program, and Organization Development* 8(4): 203-208, 1990.

Whitman, Neal and Schwenk, Thomas L. "Teaching Problem Solving." In *Surgical Teaching: Practice Makes Perfect* by Neal Whitman and Peter Lawrence. Salt Lake City: University of Utah School of Medicine, 1991.

Whitman, Neal, Weiss, Elaine, Bishop, F. Marian. *Executive Skills for Medical Faculty*. Salt Lake City: University of Utah School of Medicine, 1989.

Whitman, Neal, Weiss, Elaine, Lutz, Lawrence. *The Chief Resident as Manager*. Salt Lake City, University of Utah School of Medicine, 1988.

Wigton RS and Steinman WC. "Procedural Skills Training in the Internal Medicine Residency." *Journal of Medical Education* 59: 392-400, 1984.

Wigton RS, Patil KD, and Hoellerich VL. "The Effect of Feedback in Learning Clincal Diagnosis." *Journal of Medical Education* 61: 816-822, 1986.

Wilkerson L, Lesky L, and Medio FJ. "The Resident as Teacher During Work Rounds." *Journal of Medical Education* 61: 823-829, 1986.

Woolliscroft JO, Calhoun JG, Beauchamp C, Wolf FM, and Maxim BR. "Evaluating the Medical History: Observation Versus Write-up Review." *Journal of Medical Education* 59: 19-23, 1984.

Wray NP, Friedland JA, Ashton CM, Scheurich J, and Szollo AJ. "Characteristics of House Staff Work Rounds on Two Academic General Medicine Services." *Journal of Medical Education* 61: 893-900, 1986.

Yanoff KL and Burg FD. "Types of Medical Writing and Teaching of Writing in U.S. Medical Schools. " *Journal of Medical Education* 63: 30-37, 1988.

Yurchack PM. "A Guide to Medical Case Presentations." *Resident Staff Physician* 109-115, Sept. 1981.